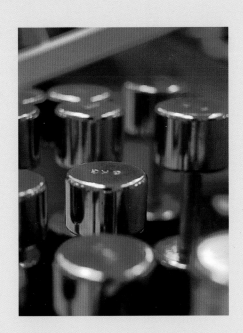

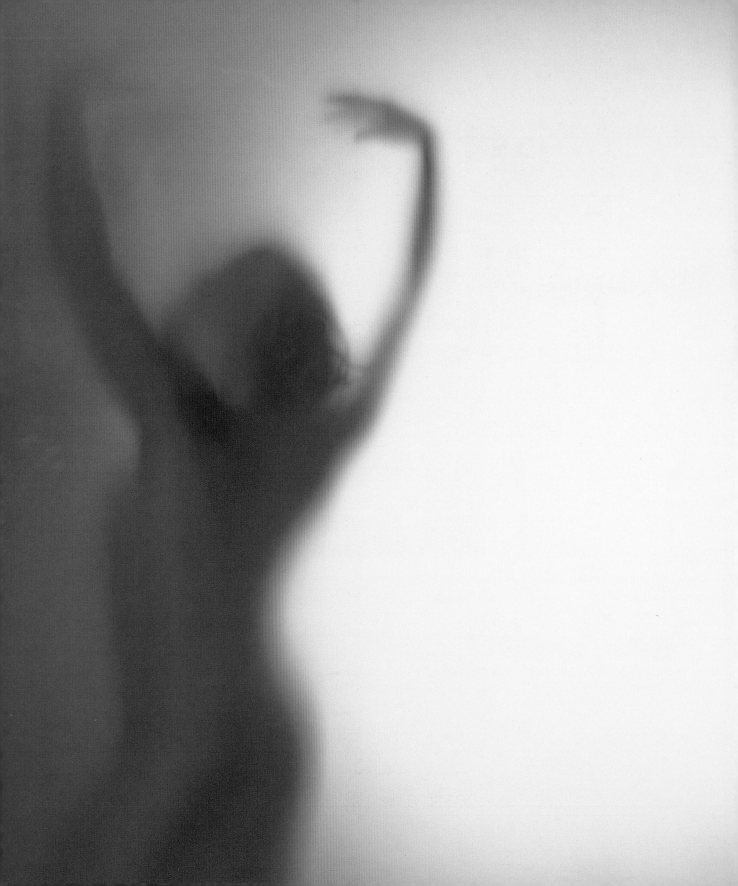

Matt Roberts

90-day
fitnessplan

Photography by Reuben Paris

A Dorling Kindersley Book

LONDON, NEW YORK, SYDNEY, DELHI, PARIS, MUNICH AND JOHANNESBURG

project editor Nasim Mawji
managing editor Gillian Roberts
managing art editor Tracey Ward
US editor Gary Werner
category publisher Mary-Clare Jerram
art director Tracy Killick
dtp designer Louise Waller
production manager Maryann Webster
photography Reuben Paris at Unit 23
food photography Janeanne Gilchrist at Unit 23

First American edition, 2001

01 02 03 04 05 10 9 8 7 6 5 4 3 2

Published in the United States by
DK Publishing, Inc.
95 Madison Avenue, New York, New York 10016

Copyright © 2001 Dorling Kindersley Limited
Text copyright © 2001 Matt Roberts Training

Always consult your doctor before starting a fitness and nutrition program if you have any health concerns.

A Cataloging-in-Publication record is available from the Library of Congress

ISBN 0-7894-7559-6

Color reproduced by Colourscan, Singapore
Printed and bound in Verona-Italy by Mondadori Printing S.p-.A

See our complete
catalog at
www.dk.com

contents

the program

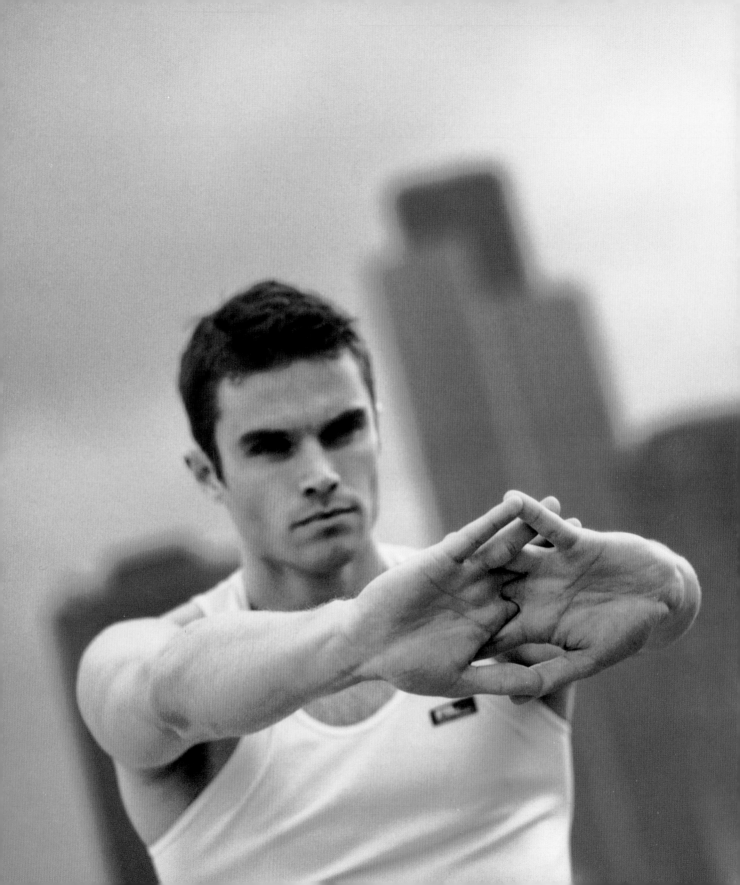

the
Matt
Roberts

A comprehensive health and fitness program needs

way

to embrace both exercise and diet, but it must also

be flexible enough to meet the needs of each

individual. Everyone has different personal goals,

but we share the common goal of wanting

a body that functions at its best.

ethos

Fitness and health have been a lifelong passion for me. I constantly strive to improve my own level of health and fitness, but as a trainer, nothing is more satisfying than helping other people to achieve their goals. I am always surprised by the extent to which a few small changes can make such a difference to the quality of people's lives.

why the program was devised

Do you feel your best? Are you happy with the shape of your body? Is your body as lean as it should or could be? Are you mentally as alert as you were? Do you spring out of bed in the morning, or do you roll out onto the floor with a thud? How motivated are you to achieve new objectives in your life? Are there things that you used to do that now seem much more difficult?

Questions like these strike a chord with most people – I found that many of my clients felt the same way. Very few people can honestly say that they think they are in great condition, and that is why I devised my program. You can feel better, physically and mentally, by making a few simple changes to the way that you eat and the way that you exercise.

Over the years I have worked with people from all kinds of different lifestyles and backgrounds, from leaders in business to musicians and actors to international athletes and, without exception, my program has worked for them. There is no such thing as a single health plan that suits everyone, so my program is flexible. After assessing your level of physical fitness, your diet, and your personality, you can tailor the program to meet your needs. My clients needed a plan that would motivate them with realistic goals without intruding on their lives; a plan that could still be followed when they couldn't get to see me. I created this program to fulfill those criteria, and that is why it has been so successful. It actually works.

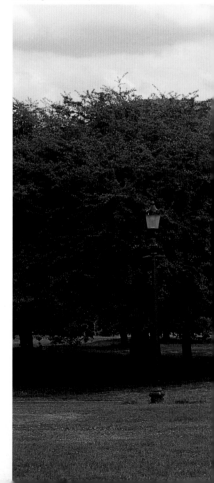

the program actually works

help your body to work efficiently

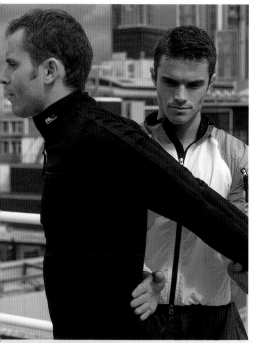

how the program developed

My program for better health has been developed after many years of guiding, training, motivating, analyzing and, of course, listening to clients. Working as a team with me, my trainers, therapists, and doctors have developed a unique insight into the way in which different people respond to changes in exercise, nutrition, and stress levels. Through medical testing we have also discovered how to use information about the body's cellular balance to improve health.

The key to feeling your best is to help your body to work as efficiently as possible. This may sound simple, but it's not always obvious what help the body needs: often we are harming our bodies without even realizing it. My revolutionary program can help, but the decision to change has to come from you.

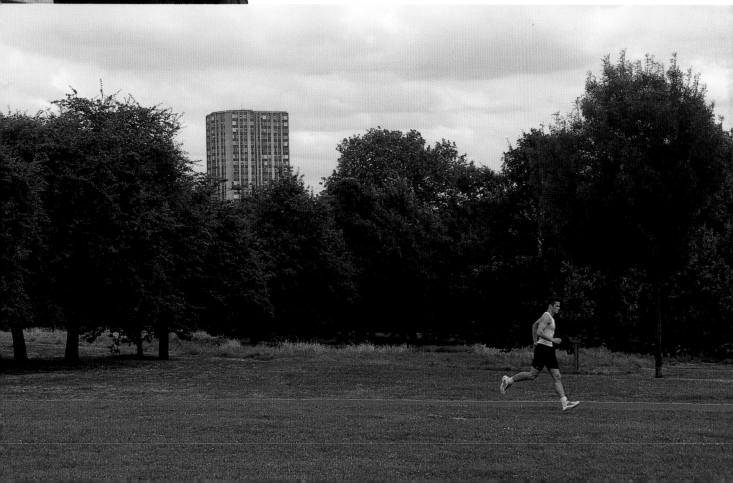

common problems

We suffer more from the effects of stress and high toxin levels in the body simply as a result of the frenetic lives that we lead. Both of these problems have a negative effect on the body and prevent it from working at optimum efficiency.

stress

There are many reasons why more people in the West are getting fatter, and obesity levels are rising faster than ever before. The obvious causes are overeating and underactivity. The less obvious cause is stress.

The stress that we know today is quite different from the stress that primitive man fighting for survival might have experienced, but the body's response to it is the same – it reacts with the "fight or flight" mechanism. When faced with danger, the body releases adrenaline into the bloodstream in order to prepare itself for a burst of intense physical activity – either to fight the danger, or to take flight and run away from it. We may not be fighting large animals these days, but the body still needs coping mechanisms, usually physical outlets, to deal with the stress it experiences.

For some people, the coping mechanism is sports or shopping; for others it may be alcohol or eating. We recognize the health implications of using alcohol to excess to cope with stress, and there are support networks in place to help people to deal with this illness. Yet more people die from eating-related conditions such as heart disease and bowel cancer than from alcohol-related illnesses. Turning to food in times of stress, and using it to help suppress problems is known as comfort eating – it is something that most of us have been guilty of at some point. It is more than just a psychological condition. Eating certain foods can trigger the body's production of serotonin, a chemical that makes you feel happy; some foods increase the levels of fat lipids

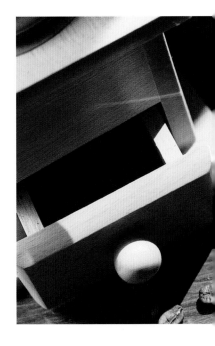

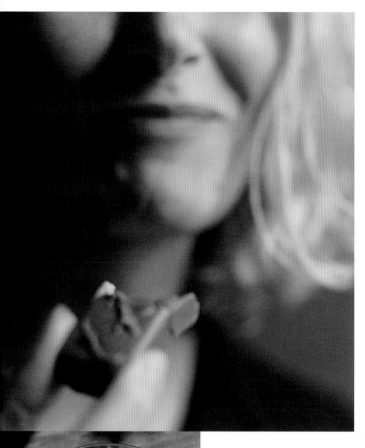

in the blood, which can have a calming effect. Sugar- and starch-based foods such as candy, chocolate, and bread all trigger the production of serotonin when you eat them. By keeping to the nutritional goals in my program, and by following the training program at the same time, you can teach your body to crave more positive highs that won't actually cause you any harm.

Improve your health and fitness and you make yourself physically and mentally stronger; as a result, you will find that you cope better with stress when you meet it.

high toxicity

We are constantly exposed to toxins: we live in a polluted world; we breathe polluted air; we eat processed and chemically treated foods. The body ingests these toxins and is often unable to rid itself of them; they then hinder its ability to function efficiently. High toxin levels in the body have been linked to lethargy, reduced immune function, poor natural detoxification, weight gain, and even heart disease.

My medical team and I run tests on all of our clients to assess how efficiently their bodies are functioning. We call this assessing their biological terrain, the internal environment of the body. The healthier your internal environment, the better equipped your body is to deal with stress, fight disease, maintain energy levels, keep itself healthy and, crucially, prevent the buildup of toxins.

My program aims to detoxify the body initially, then to help you to reduce the amount of toxins that you put into your body. It will help you to create a healthy biological terrain by controlling stress through exercise and by encouraging you to eat wholesome, healthy foods. If you also drink plenty of water and reduce your intake of processed foods, you will feel the positive benefits of the program in no time at all.

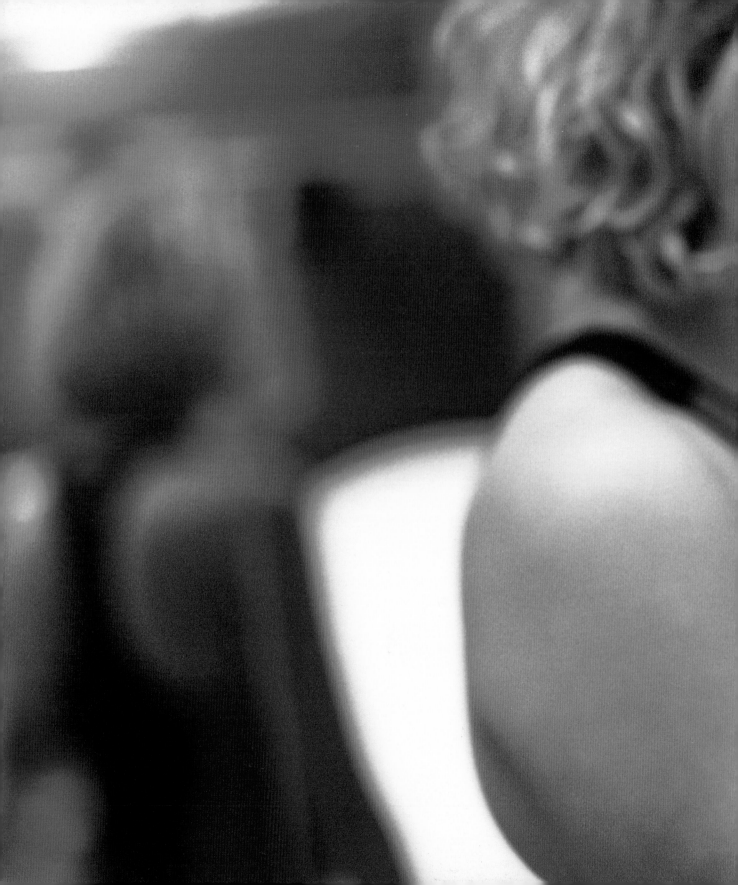

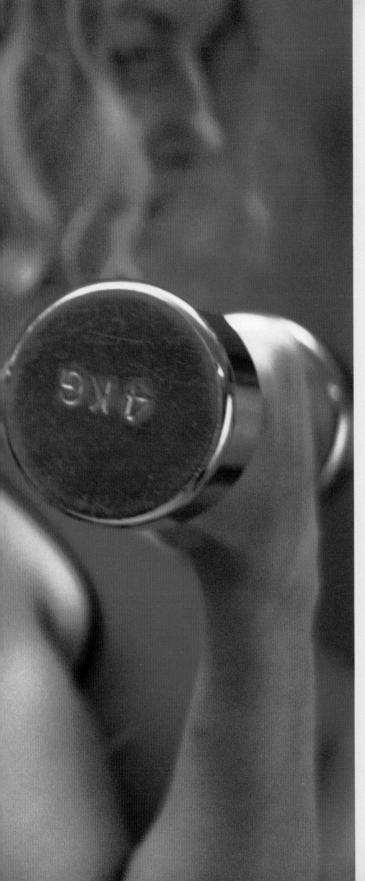

what is fitness?

Your level of fitness has a direct effect on your

quality of life – it is keeping you vital and alive.

A good level of health and fitness means you can

fulfill your potential, both physically and mentally.

By looking after your body and challenging it, you

empower yourself rather than limit your options.

popular myths

People absorb information about exercise and diet from many different sources, but it is not always correct. It is time to dispel some of the popular myths that surround health and fitness. Here are four of the most common ones that I come across.

muscle turns to fat when you stop exercising

This is based on the fear that all the effort that you have put into your exercise regime will have been wasted if you stop exercising. However, because muscle and fat are completely different body tissues, it is physically impossible for one to become the other. It is true that if you stop exercising you will gain some fat, but this is because your muscles decrease in size if they are not sufficiently challenged. With less muscle, your body is less efficient at burning energy, so you will have a tendency to gain fat.

all fat in your diet is bad

People go to great lengths to eliminate fat from their diets in the belief that it will prevent their body from accumulating more fat. What people don't realize is that fat plays a very important role in the body, and without it, your body would suffer. You need to distinguish between good fats, such as olive oil, which are liquid at room temperature, and bad fats, such as butter, which are solid at room temperature *(see pages 18–19)*.

if I exercise with weights, I will get bulky

Many people fear that weight training will make them overmuscular. But it is actually very

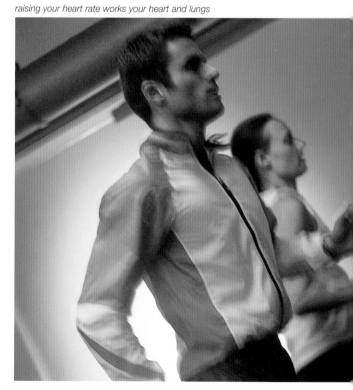

raising your heart rate works your heart and lungs

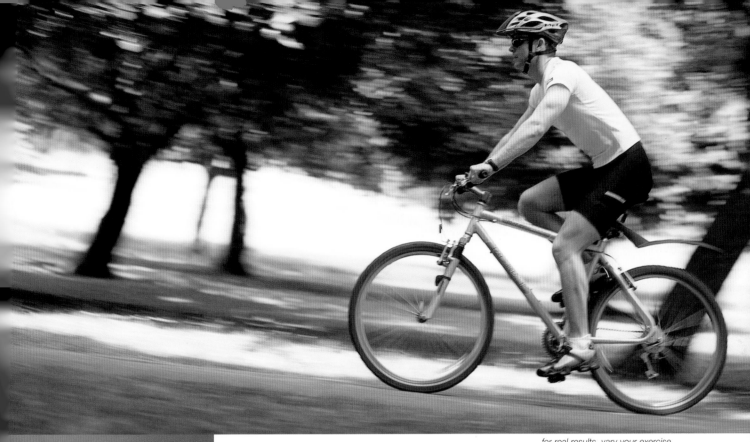

for real results, vary your exercise

difficult to create muscle tissue. The short-term accumulation of body fluids within the tissues of the muscle can make you feel as though you have gained muscle but, in actual fact, you haven't. To build muscle mass, you need to be constantly overloading the muscles, or testing them. Provided you vary your exercise routine and you test the body in different ways, weight training will not make you bulky.

doing yoga and Pilates is enough to keep me fit

Both yoga and Pilates are excellent forms of exericse. They encourage muscle flexibility and good posture and can have very positive mental benefits. However, you should never just run, just lift weights, or just cycle. True fitness is about challenging every part of your body in many ways, and there is no single form of exercise that can do this on its own. To see real results, you need to raise your heart rate to an appropriate level three to four times a week and vary your exercise to work your heart, lungs, muscles, and internal organs.

15

the facts

Diet and fitness have been hot topics for years. "Experts" are forever trying to sell us different theories and fads about attaining the body beautiful. This is where I set the record straight.

resistance training

Whether you want to lose weight, gain weight, develop stronger bones or burn fat, resistance training, or weight training, will help you – it is the key to your program. Muscle burns the most energy in your body, and the more you use it, the more energy it burns. If you exercise regularly doing a purely aerobic activity such as running or swimming, for example, you may find that you reach a point where you are unable to lose weight or burn fat. This is likely to be because you are not pushing yourself sufficiently. It may sound ridiculous because of the amount of effort that you put into your exercise, but you may be overlooking a small aspect of your routine that could make a crucial difference.

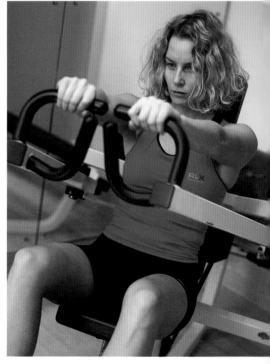

resistance training – the key

That small aspect is muscle utilization, or the degree to which you use your muscles. Muscle is made up of many thousands of tiny muscle fibers that become dormant when not used. Going about day-to-day tasks, you probably use about 40 percent of your muscle fibers – if you were to use 100 percent, you would burn energy at 100 percent efficiency. The fewer muscle fibers you use, the easier it is for your body to gradually gain weight because it is not working to its full capability. My program challenges your muscles without encouraging them to grow substantially. Resistance training can also raise your basal metabolic rate (BMR), the rate at which you burn energy to keep functioning and alive, which means that you burn more calories while simply sitting still.

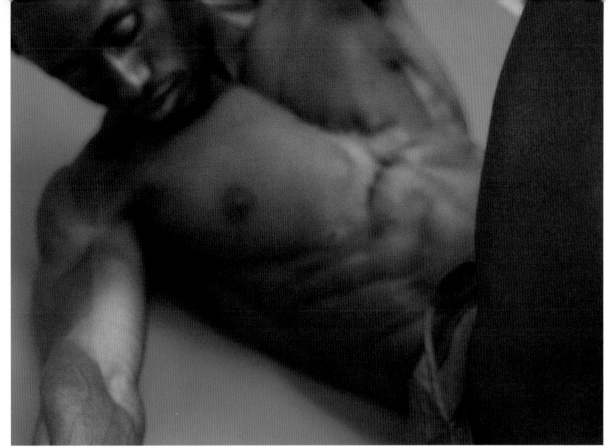

my program challenges the body

aerobic training

Once you have begun challenging your body with resistance training, an aerobic training routine is the next step. Aerobic training increases the body's oxygen consumption, which helps your body to burn energy and strengthens your heart. Aerobic training is key to optimum fitness.

My program tests you in different ways: from Constant Pace Training, which involves training intensively for long periods to build endurance, to Interval Training, which builds cardiovascular strength and is also one of the most effective ways of burning calories.

To get the most out of aerobic training, you need to work within your optimum training zone. Calculate this by first determining your maximum heart rate (MHR): assume that your MHR when you are born is 220 and that every year your heart rate reduces by one, so your MHR = 220 minus your age. So, if you are 40, your MHR is 180 beats per minute (BPM). For your optimum training zone, see page 43.

overall body function

With any health and fitness program it is important to treat the whole body. Trying to tackle one problem area does not work. If, for example, you are concerned about your thighs and concentrate all your efforts on that one area, the effect will be that they become out of proportion with the rest of your body, so aggravating the problem. Any program must address the needs of the inner and outer body through a combination of diet and exercise that works the heart, lungs, and muscles.

good fats, bad fats

Most diets tell you that to lose weight you have to eliminate or at least reduce the amount of fat in your diet, but they miss the point. Your body positively needs fat to live; in fact a healthy diet should consist of no less than 15–20 percent fat. This may sound like a lot, but fats are essential for the efficient functioning of muscles, healthy blood, good digestion, even healthy hair and skin – in fact, for most of the body's processes. I am not saying that all fat is good, though, and you certainly can't allow chips, fries, and burgers to make up 20 percent of your diet. What you need to know is that fats come in good and bad forms. The bad fats are animal fats such as butter, the fat around red meat, and hydrogenated fats such as margarine and cooking fats commonly used in baking and as binding agents in cheap processed foods. The simple way to identify them is that they are usually solid at room temperature. Bad fats have been linked with heart disease, strokes, cancer, and many other illnesses, and for this reason should be reduced to a minimum in your diet.

Olive oil and the fats in fish, nuts, seeds, and grains are good fats, known as essential fatty acids. Good fats are generally liquid at room temperature. This doesn't mean that just because some fats are good, you can drown your food in olive oil and not gain weight. Good fats are still fats and what the body cannot use, it stores as excess calories. Do remember that nuts contain good fat. So many people avoid nuts because they think they are fattening; in fact they are highly nutritious and, eaten in moderation (a handful a day, for example) they make a terrific alternative to snacks such as chocolate and cookies.

the diet-only approach

Diet is an important part of the program, but it is only one part. You cannot make substantial changes to your body through diet alone. The most effective way to lose weight – and keep it off – is through a combined approach of regular exercise and healthy diet. The majority of people who follow a diet-only program gain the weight they have lost, and in many cases more, within six months of stopping the diet. Dieting doesn't burn calories, it just slows your body down. Every time you slow down, the body finds it more difficult to return to normal, and as a result, it functions less efficiently and you gain weight. Follow the program's nutritional guidelines; but remember, for lasting results, you need to follow the exercise plan as well.

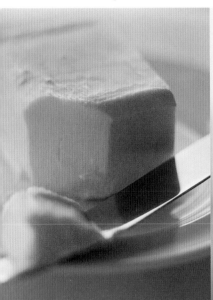

butter – enjoy it just occasionally

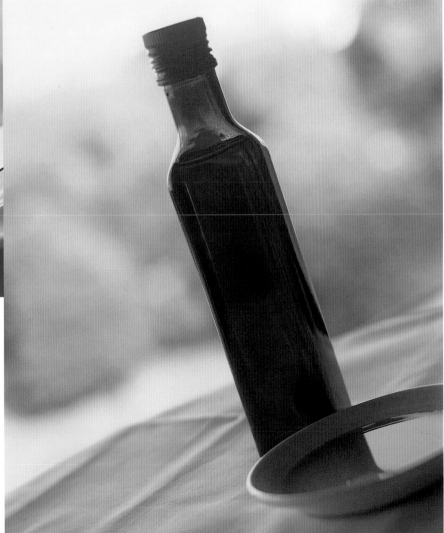

olive oil is a good fat

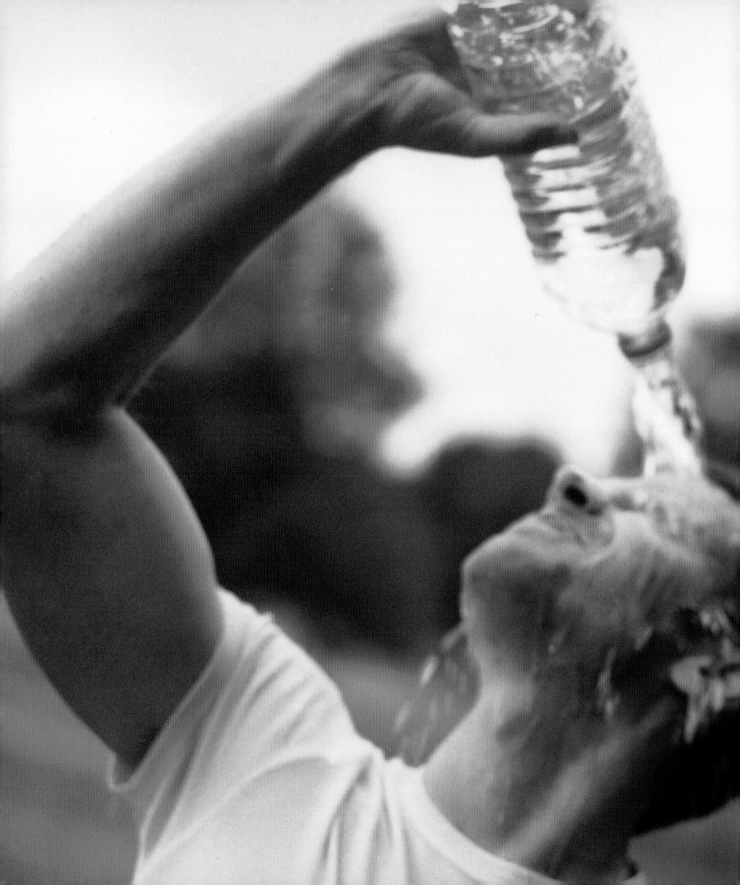

why
detox?

When toxins build up in your cells, your body

functions less efficiently. The symptoms can

be anything from lethargy and weight gain to

headaches and irritability. A diet and lifestyle

that aid detoxification will help to control and

reduce toxin buildup and boost energy levels.

body processes

The human body is a truly amazing machine. It can cope with situations and problems more competently than any computer. Sometimes this machine falters, but it signals when it is unable to perform at optimum efficiency; we need to listen to and understand these signals. Here I look at how the body responds to problems and how you can help your own body to overcome them.

when did you last feel fantastic?

Very few people can honestly say that they feel fantastic. You may not even remember the last time you really felt healthy and at one with yourself. You don't suddenly gain weight or suddenly feel lethargic – the extra weight creeps up on you without your noticing, and you just might not feel as energetic as you once did.

Modern living encourages us to be lazy. If you threw away your television remote control and changed channels manually instead, with the extra energy you expended, you could, in theory, lose about two pounds in a year. It doesn't sound like much, but with all the labor-saving devices that make our lives easier – from elevators and escalators to electric windows – we give our bodies the opportunity to be less active. The less active you are, the more the body slows down and the less incentive there is to eat and drink healthily. Your toxin levels rise, and as a result you feel even more lethargic.

Don't make excuses for yourself. It's not difficult to reverse the downward spiral. If you think you don't have enough time to follow a health program, you are just the type of person who has the most to gain from it because it is your system that is probably under the most strain from your lifestyle. Don't think that you are too old to start exercising either. You will find that you have strengths that a younger person may not have.

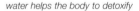

water helps the body to detoxify

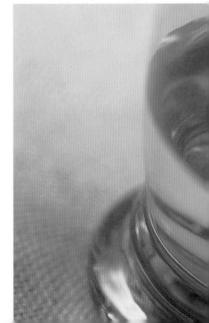

are you at one with yourself?

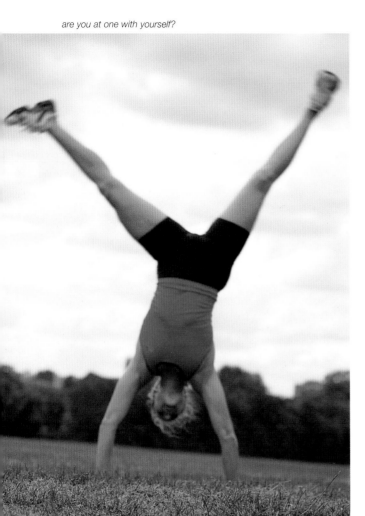

toxic buildup

It is very likely that over the years your body has accumulated toxins – poor diet, stress, and inactivity all contribute to their buildup. You may have experienced lethargy or poor digestion, or found that you can't lose weight or have difficulty concentrating. They are all indicators that your body is not functioning as efficiently as it could be, and the most common cause is toxic buildup in your body's cells.

We constantly expose our bodies to toxins. Most of us have eaten processed foods, inhaled cigarette smoke (whether passively or actively), and drunk alcohol – it can be difficult to avoid doing these things. Each time you do, you reduce your body's ability to function efficiently. The more you expose your body to toxins, the less efficient it becomes at ridding itself of them and the more you are likely to suffer as a consequence.

Dehydration is to blame for many of the symptoms that people associate with feeling unwell. Your body is between 60 and 65 percent water, and to help it defend itself against the onslaught of toxins, you have to keep it adequately hydrated. You need to drink between one and a half and two quarts of water a day, possibly even more to counteract the diuretic effects of tea, coffee, alcohol, and sugary drinks. Research has proven that mental agility can be improved by reducing toxin levels in your system; some research has even suggested that people who avoid processed foods and get regular exercise are more successful in the workplace than those who do not.

High toxin levels in your body may increase your vulnerability to viruses, infection, and other more serious illnesses. Following a program of detoxification can help your body to function more efficiently.

lethargy

Many of us accept lethargy as a normal consequence of our fast-moving, stressful lifestyles. We all feel tired from time to time, whether as a result of lack of sleep or stress, but these periods of tiredness should not last long. Feeling persistently fatigued can put physical and mental strain on your body.

One of the most common causes of lethargy is not eating properly. People diet excessively and deprive themselves of food or simply don't eat enough nutrient-rich foods to fuel the body sufficiently. This can then be compounded by eating too many processed foods, which tend to be low in nutrients. This slows the body down and can result in a weakened immune system, disturbed sleep, and poor concentration. The body becomes less efficient at ridding itself of toxins and deficient in essential nutrients. Noticeable results are dry or blemished skin and unhealthy hair. It can also have a damaging effect on our bones.

Another increasingly common reason for lethargy is food intolerance (*see page 26*). If you eat large quantities of certain foods, the body can develop an intolerance to them and begin to produce toxins as it has difficulty digesting them. Toxins inhibit the cells' ability to generate energy. They can build up as a result of stress, poor diet, lack of exercise and dehydration, and leave you feeling listless and lethargic.

poor digestion

It is not just the food that we eat that gives us energy. It is how efficient our body is at breaking it down and extracting nutrients from it. Digestion starts in the mouth. Often people simply eat too quickly without chewing their food thoroughly enough. Saliva starts the digestive process and breaks down food as it is chewed. Once swallowed, enzymes in the digestive system break it down further and the body begins to absorb nutrients from it. If food has not been chewed properly, the body is less able to extract nutrients from it, and as a result, may be deprived of the energy it needs to function healthily.

Processed foods and foods manufactured with artificial pesticides and preservatives may not be as good at maintaining a balance of healthy bacteria in the digestive system as fresh foods in their natural state.

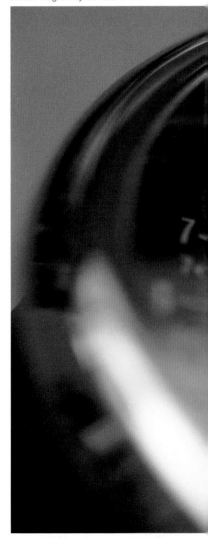

excess weight may be hard to lose

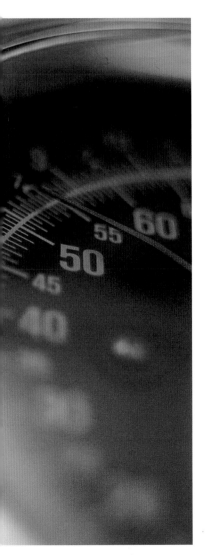

weight retention

A common complaint is not being able to lose stubborn excess fat, no matter what you do. There can be a number of different reasons for this, and although food intolerance (*see page 26*) and dehydration (*see page 22*) can be factors, the main causes are unsuitable exercise regimes and yo-yo dieting, both of which lower the metabolic rate.

Many people attempt to burn fat by spending hours on the treadmill or step machine, for example, but this is not an effective long-term strategy for weight loss. Aerobic exercise is very important – it burns calories, strengthens the heart and lungs, and reduces cholesterol levels – but it is not your only weapon in the fight against fat.

Aim to increase your metabolic rate, that is, the rate at which your body burns energy, and therefore calories and fat. The more toned your muscles, the higher your metabolic rate. Although aerobic training will have some toning effect on the legs, it won't actually build the important energy-burning muscles of the upper body. You can achieve this only through resistance training.

Ensure that you eat enough nutrient-rich food to sustain you through aerobic exercise. Exercising when your energy levels are low can cause muscle wastage and reduce metabolic rate.

By combining aerobic training and isolated resistance work, as I do in my program, you can improve muscle tone, increase metabolic rate, and strengthen the heart and lungs. Even when at rest, the body will burn calories at a higher rate, which means that losing extra fat and maintaining your ideal body shape will be much easier for you.

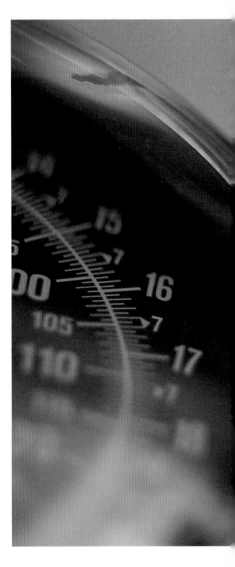

yo-yo dieting

The effect of crash diet after crash diet, without exercise, may be weight loss, but the weight is muscle tissue as well as fat. Metabolic rate is linked to the amount of muscle you have, so if you constantly go on diets that lower your muscle mass, you constantly lower your metabolic rate. The inevitable consequence of this is that after the diet you gain weight more easily because your metabolic rate is so low. The more you crash diet, the more muscle tissue is reduced and the lower the metabolic rate becomes. This goes on until it is almost impossible to maintain a normal weight.

Crash dieting is not a healthy or a permanent way to lose weight. Fueling the body with nutrient-rich food and exercising to increase the metabolic rate through improving muscle tone is the most effective way to achieve long-term weight loss.

food intolerances

It is estimated that up to as many as 90 percent of people suffer food intolerances that affect their lives in some way or other. Symptoms can range from lethargy, headaches, asthma, and eczema to arthritis, difficulty losing weight, and obesity.

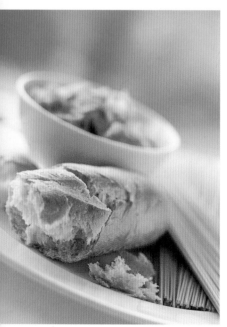

eat fewer wheat products

An intolerance to a food is quite different from an allergy to it. With a food allergy, the body has a dramatic chemical reaction to a food that it cannot deal with. The manifestation can be anything from an immediate skin rash to inflammation of the air passage, which, in severe cases, can restrict breathing. Nuts and seafood are the most common food allergens.

Food intolerance occurs when the body finds it difficult to digest a food and produces toxic by-products as it attempts to break it down. This can result in a buildup of toxins which can then impair the immune system and affect energy production in the body. An excessive buildup of toxins can slow the body down and result in any one or more of the *intolerances to wheat and yeast are common*

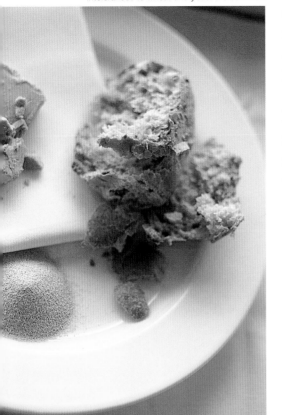

symptoms mentioned earlier. A reaction to a specific food intolerance can build up over a long period of time, but an allergic reaction to a food is likely to be immediate and can be quite violent.

You can have a permanent intolerance to a food. If your body has always found a particular food difficult to digest, it probably always will. Dairy products, shrimp, and cashew nuts are common examples; and in such cases, identifying the food and reducing your intake of it, or eliminating it from your diet altogether, can have a profound and positive effect on your energy levels and immune system.

It is also possible for your body to develop an intolerance to a food. This often happens with foods such as wheat, which you could easily eat – as cereal, bread, or pasta, for example – at almost every meal. Our overreliance on it can cause the body to produce extra toxins as a reaction to eating too much of it. Permanent elimination of a food to which you have developed an intolerance is not necessary, but it may be beneficial to give your body a temporary break from it.

I have reduced the intake of the two most common offenders – wheat and dairy – as part of the program's nutritional goals. The other common causes of food intolerance are tomatoes, shellfish, yeast, peanuts and cashew nuts, artificial colorings, food stabilizers and additives, sweeteners, and alcohol. Food intolerances differ from one person to the next, and reducing your intake of these things and foods that you feel do not agree with you is a good way to detect intolerances.

The results can be amazing. I have seen arthritis sufferers reduce their pain significantly in no time at all; a client suffering from lethargy told me that she felt incredible for the first time in years after only eight weeks.

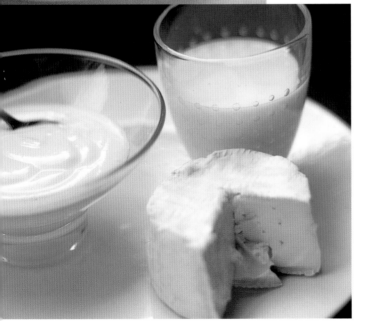

dairy products can be difficult to digest

27

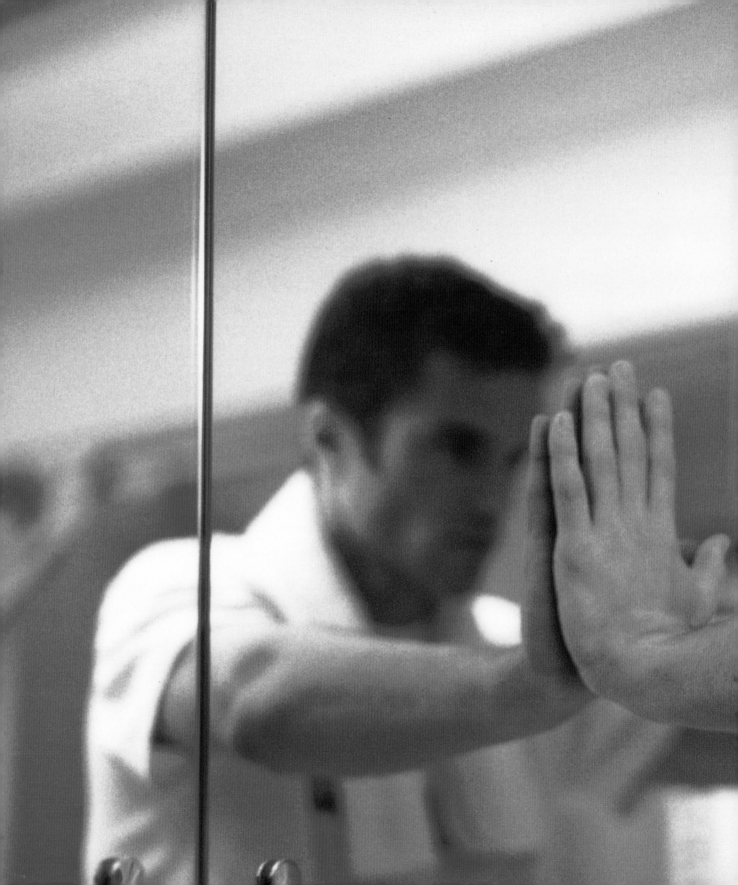

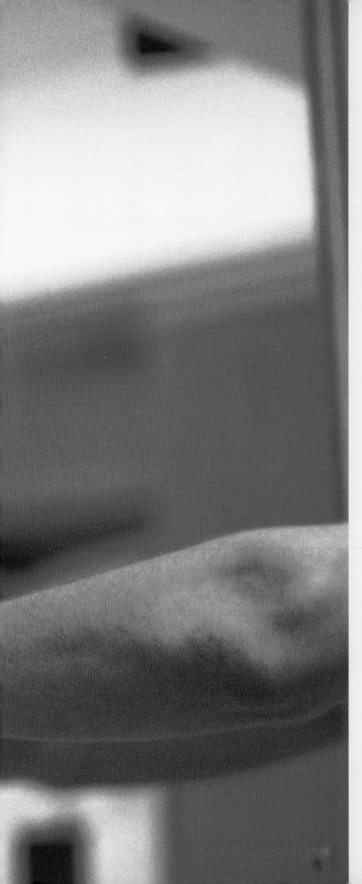

where
are you
n o w ?

Your fitness level, diet, personality, and ability to

manage stress all affect your general health. The

questionnaires that follow assess all of these factors

and will help you to tailor the program to meet

your personal needs.

physical questionnaire

The series of tests below assesses your cardiovascular fitness, strength, flexibility, and body proportions. The answers will enable you to evaluate your current level of physical fitness and help you to pinpoint areas that need work. Be honest and record your true scores. For the results, see page 137.

1 Body Mass Index (BMI) evaluation

This assesses your weight in relation to your height and gives an indication of how healthy your current body shape is.

Divide your weight in kilograms by your height in meters squared (1lb = 0.45 kg 1ft = 30.48 cm).

So, if you weigh 52 kg and are 1.72 m tall, first calculate your height squared (1.72 x 1.72 = 2.96), then divide 52 by 2.96 to give you a BMI of 18.

(a) Male: 26.1 or more
Female: 26.1 or more

(b) Male: 21–26
Female: 21–26

(c) Male: up to 20.9
Female: up to 20.9

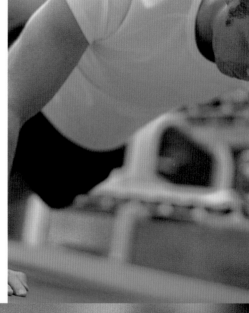

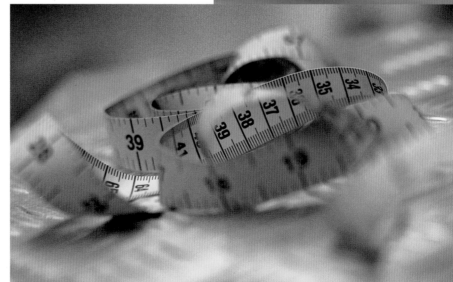

2 One-minute push-up test

This tests your upper body strength.

Do as many full push-ups or easier half push-ups *(see page 82)* as you can in one minute. Whichever you choose, always use the same push-up to test in the future. If you cannot do a full minute of push-ups, count the number you complete before your technique suffers.

Full push-ups

(a) Male: 9 or less
Female: 4 or less

(b) Male: 10–30
Female: 5–15

(c) Male: 31 or more
Female: 16 or more

Half push-ups

(a) Male: 29 or less
Female: 24 or less

(b) Male: 30–50
Female: 25–40

(c) Male: 51 or more
Female: 41 or more

3 One-minute crunch test

This tests the strength of your abdominals, or stomach muscles.

Do as many basic crunches *(see page 98)* as you can in one minute. Stop and start if you need to, but keep your technique correct.

(a) Male: 24 or less
Female: 24 or less

(b) Male: 25–45
Female: 25–45

(c) Male: 46 or more
Female: 46 or more

4 Sit and reach test

This assesses your spine and leg area flexibility.

Sit with your back against a wall and your legs together, extended in front of you. Reach forward and measure how far down your legs your fingertips touch.

(a) Thighs

(b) Bottom of knee cap

(c) Shin and beyond

5 Three-minute step test

This tests your cardiovascular fitness.

Use a step or bench that is 16 inches (40 cm) high and step up and down at a rate of 30 steps per minute. Do step ups *(see page 97)* for 3 minutes, breathing normally throughout. Stop and take your pulse for 15 seconds *(see pages 42–3)*, then multiply the figure by 4 to give your number of beats per minute.

(a) Male: 157 or more
Female: 167 or more

(b) Male: 131–156
Female: 141–166

(c) Male: 120–130
Female: 128–140

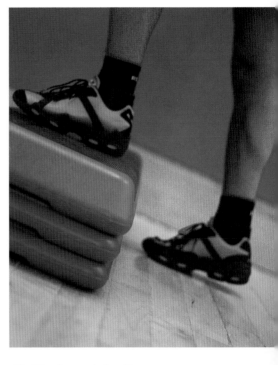

6 Hip-to-waist ratio

This test assesses your body shape and fat distribution.

Measure the hips (just below the top of the pelvis), then measure your waist (over your belly button). Divide your waist measurement by your hip measurement (you can use either metric or imperial measurements).

(a) Male: above 0.95
Female: above 0.86

(b) Male: 0.81–0.94
Female: 0.71–0.85

(c) Male: below 0.8
Female: below 0.7

nutrition questionnaire

This questionnaire tests how healthy your diet is, how well your body responds to it, and how effective your digestion is. It also assesses your body's acid/alkaline balance, which can affect your energy levels and general health. For the results, see page 138.

1 How much water do you drink each day?

(a) Less than 2 cups (½ liter)
(b) 2–4 cups (½–1 liter)
(c) More than 4 cups (1 liter)

2 How many cups of coffee or tea do you drink each day?

(a) More than 4 cups
(b) 2–4 cups
(c) 1 cup

3 How many sugary or carbonated drinks do you normally have each day?

(a) More than 4
(b) 2–4
(c) 1

4 How many pieces of fruit do you eat each day?

(a) 0–1
(b) 1–3
(c) More than 3

5 How many portions of fresh vegetables do you eat each week?

(a) 2–4
(b) 4–7
(c) more than 7

6 How often do you eat breakfast?

(a) Never
(b) Sometimes
(c) Always

7 How often do you eat after 8pm?

(a) Regularly
(b) Occasionally
(c) Never

8 How many of your daily meals contain red meat?

(a) 2 meals
(b) 1 meal
(c) 0 meals

9 How many of your daily meals contain wheat in any form? (*Bread, pasta, noodles, cereals, cookies, etc.*)

(a) 3 meals
(b) 2 meals
(c) 1 meal

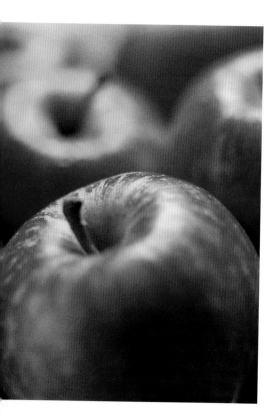

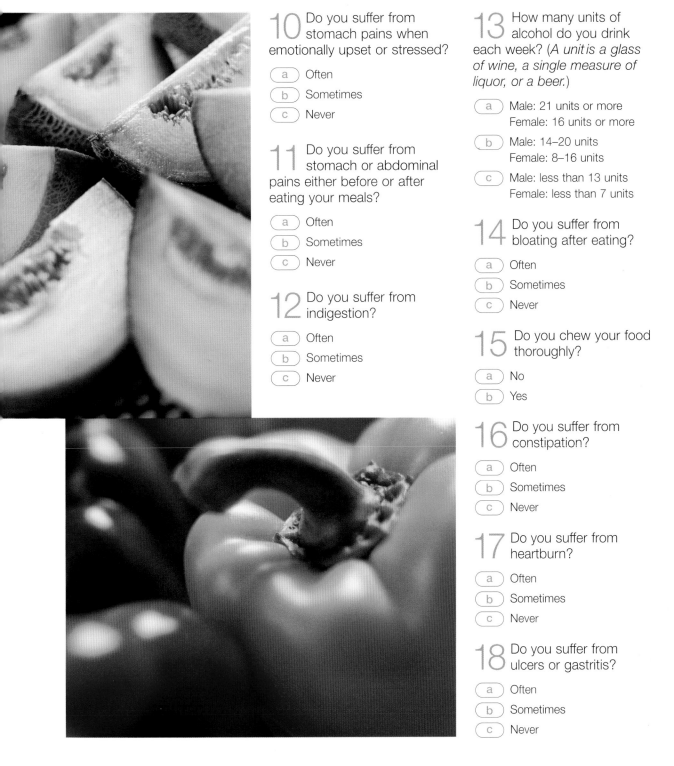

10 Do you suffer from stomach pains when emotionally upset or stressed?

(a) Often
(b) Sometimes
(c) Never

11 Do you suffer from stomach or abdominal pains either before or after eating your meals?

(a) Often
(b) Sometimes
(c) Never

12 Do you suffer from indigestion?

(a) Often
(b) Sometimes
(c) Never

13 How many units of alcohol do you drink each week? (*A unit is a glass of wine, a single measure of liquor, or a beer.*)

(a) Male: 21 units or more
Female: 16 units or more
(b) Male: 14–20 units
Female: 8–16 units
(c) Male: less than 13 units
Female: less than 7 units

14 Do you suffer from bloating after eating?

(a) Often
(b) Sometimes
(c) Never

15 Do you chew your food thoroughly?

(a) No
(b) Yes

16 Do you suffer from constipation?

(a) Often
(b) Sometimes
(c) Never

17 Do you suffer from heartburn?

(a) Often
(b) Sometimes
(c) Never

18 Do you suffer from ulcers or gastritis?

(a) Often
(b) Sometimes
(c) Never

personality questionnaire

The extensive research we have carried out with our clients has enabled us to identify characteristics of the two basic personality types. We have discovered clear links between personality and stress management, toxin levels, and digestive problems. For the results, see page 139.

1 Do you regularly have difficulty sleeping?
(a) Yes
(b) No

2 Do you make decisions quickly?
(a) Yes
(b) No

3 Does time-wasting annoy you?
(a) Yes
(b) No

4 Do you have a tendency to take on more than you can handle?
(a) Yes
(b) No

5 Is time always against you?
(a) Yes
(b) No

6 Do you spend time relaxing and pampering yourself?
(a) Yes
(b) No

7 Do you feel that your skills are suited to the job you do?
(a) Yes
(b) No

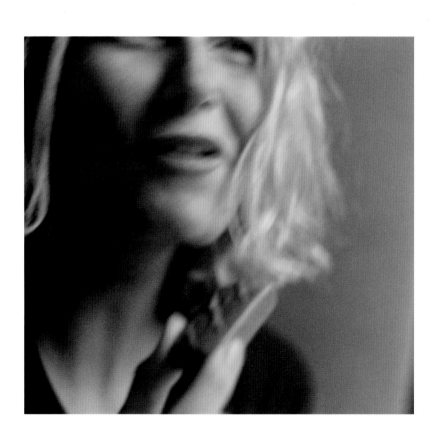

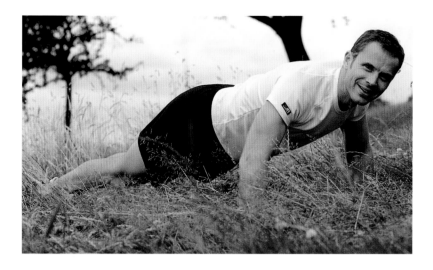

8 Do you feel that you have support from your family and friends?

- (a) Yes
- (b) No

9 Do you feel that your position at work is constantly threatened?

- (a) Yes
- (b) No

10 Do you have a long attention span?

- (a) Yes
- (b) No

11 Do you bottle up problems?

- (a) Yes
- (b) No

12 Are you liable to mood swings?

- (a) Yes
- (b) No

13 Do you find that alcohol helps you relax after a hard day?

- (a) Yes
- (b) No

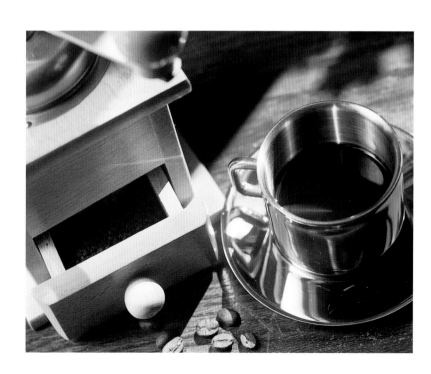

setting your goals

If you don't know where you are going, how will you know when you have arrived? Most diets and exercise programs fail because of inadequate or unrealistic goal setting. Focus on your short-term goals and your ultimate long-term goals will fall into place.

staying on course

Approach your goal setting in the same way as you would go about building a house. You know what you are going to build, and you have an image of the final outcome in mind, but you have to plan each individual stage of the building according to short-term targets.

set realistic goals

Write your own list of long- and short-term goals. They will become your manifesto over the next 90 days. Keep your goals in mind and never stray from them. Write them as if you were writing your own personal self-help guide.

There may be moments in the program when you start to drift and lose sight of your goals. At these moments it will be most important for you to have your written goals to refer to, to remind you of your motivation. Indeed, this stage of the program may prove to be one of the most challenging for you. You may be aware that you want to make changes, but now you must quantify them and set a date for their completion. It may help to think back to when you were at your fittest. Then you can set achievable goals that are specific to you. These goals are the basis of your overall plan and are the fundamental reason you have decided to embark on my program. Use them to your advantage.

long-term goals

If you already have a long-term goal in mind, write it down. That goal is your destination point – the point in your "house building" at which

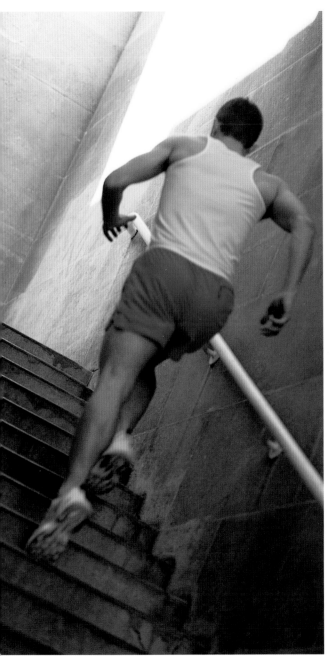

be proud of what you achieve

you can get rid of the builders and be proud of what you have achieved. If you don't have a goal in mind, think of one, and make it specific. If you want to change clothes size, what will your new clothes size be? If you want to lose weight, how much will you lose? If you want to run a marathon, which one, where, and when? Be specific, and more importantly, be realistic. If your goal is to look like a supermodel, you will probably be disappointed. You can set yourself a difficult goal, but choose it carefully and make sure that it is an achievable goal, even if difficult. It is the key to your motivation and should be something that is important to you.

Write your long-term goal down as a promise to yourself. Treat it like your mission statement; write it as if you were making a contract with yourself: "I (state your name) will achieve (state your goal) by (state your date)." Attach a reward to the goal. "On achieving (your goal), I will (state your reward)."

You might reward yourself by doing something with your newfound fitness. You might want to shop for the clothes that you thought wouldn't fit. It is your choice, but your greatest reward is the change to yourself. Choose whatever motivates you personally. You may even want to put in a penalty clause: "Should I not achieve (state your goal), I will (state your penalty)." For example, you could promise to take over a household chore that you dislike doing, for a month.

Focus on your long-term goal. Aim for it and keep it in mind. Once you have achieved it, you can be very proud indeed.

short-term goals

Your short-term goals are crucial because they lead you to your ultimate goal. No matter how minor or trivial they might seem, they still make a difference to your overall result. You might want to ask for assistance from the people around you – they can often help to keep you on track.

short-term goals

Once you have set your long-term goal, start thinking about the short-term goals that will help you to achieve it. I set a number of diet and exercise goals at the start of each phase in the program; they are some of your short-term goals. The goals are relatively easy to achieve: drinking eight cups (two liters) of water every day or exercising four times a week, for example.

During the first two phases of the program short-term goals are set every three weeks. This may be when you make the biggest changes to your lifestyle, but this gives you enough time to adjust to them and to work them into your routine. Each time you are set new goals, add them to your previous set to build an overall list. The final phase takes two weeks. Use the last day of the program to assess how you have done against the goals you set. Be realistic and reward yourself for good performance. If you have not achieved your goals, it is time to set a new plan of action.

Set your own short-term goals by looking at each of the phases and make a note of the areas that you feel will require a particular effort from you to change them. Once you combine the goals that I give you with the goals that you devise yourself you should have about four or five for each phase of the book.

With your short-term goals in place, you have the foundation for all of your future achievements. See them as a strategy for your life plan.

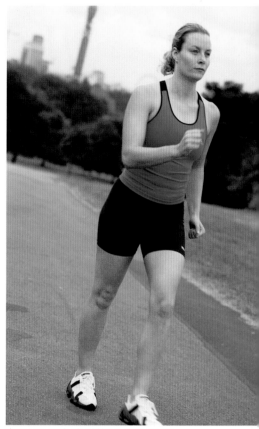

short-term goals should be easy to achieve

external influences

One of the important elements of a successful health program is the support network of people that you have around you – they are your external influences. You are probably going to be making some significant changes to your lifestyle, and there will be days when you feel tired or don't feel like exercising, or when you want to eat or drink contrary to the program. Having supportive people around you is exceptionally helpful because they can help to keep you on track. Tell the people around you what you are doing. If they know how important the program is to you, they will be more likely to help you through any bad moments. They can probably help you with your short-term goals, especially if you see them every day. You never know – you may be able to persuade your partner or a friend to join you.

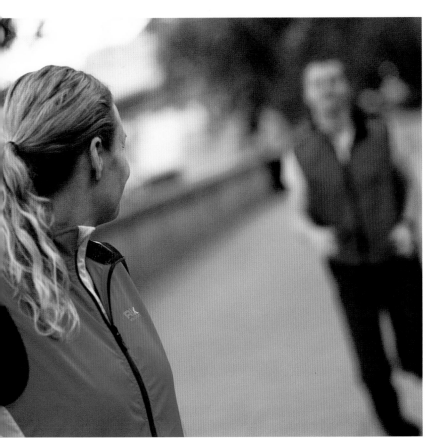

you might persuade your partner or a friend to join you

internal influences

You also have an internal sphere of influence. They are the people that you consider to be your role models or mentors. Are these people the epitome of good health, or have they seen better days? Think of people who have a level of health and fitness that you aspire to and that you feel you could attain.

If the people around you do not consider good health and fitness to be important, you may find that you have to be even more determined to focus on the challenges ahead. You may not be able to avoid these people entirely, so refer to your written goals to remind you of your motivation and determination to stay on track.

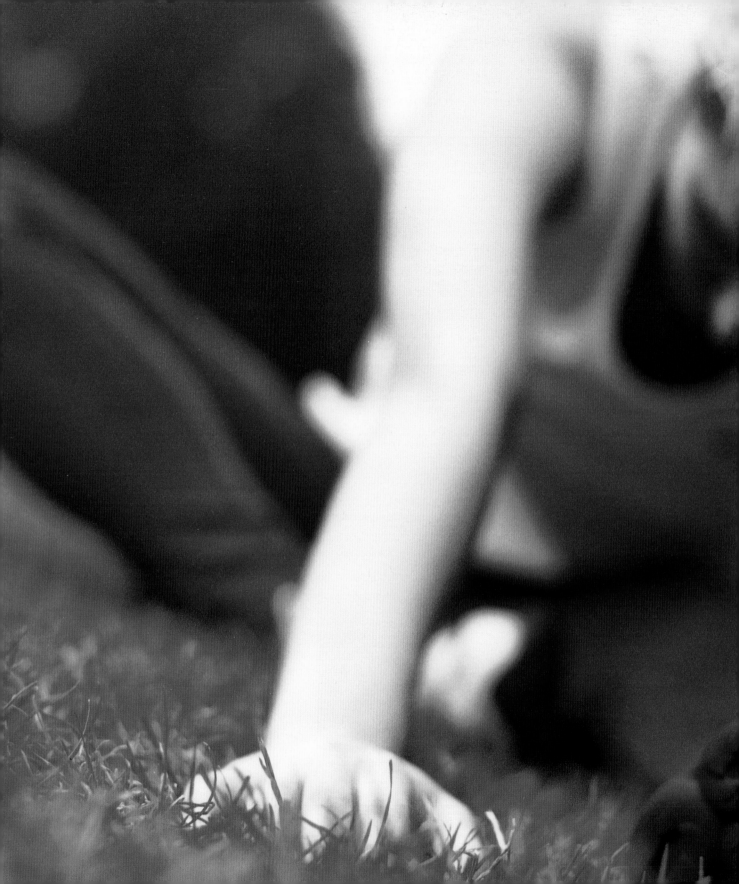

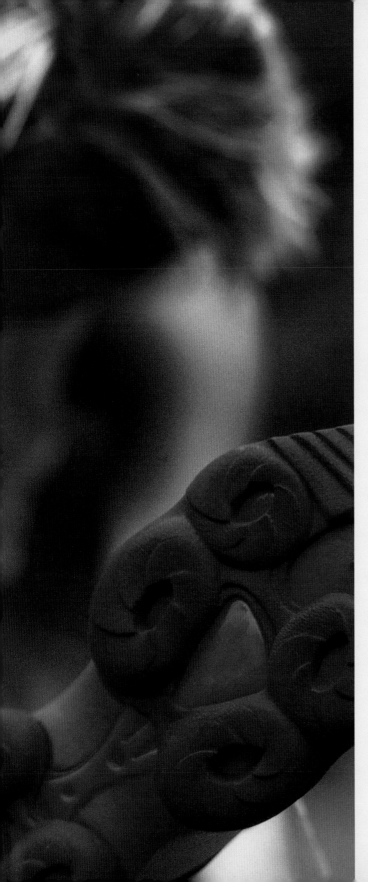

the
basics

To make significant changes to your body, you

need to understand how it works and how it will

respond to the program's nutritional goals and

training techniques. Here are the basics of fitness,

from the optimum level to work your heart and

lungs to how far to test your muscles.

aerobic training

A good level of aerobic fitness has been proven to guard against heart disease and stress-related disorders. Aerobic training is an essential part of any fitness program.

heart rate training zones

Aerobic simply means "with oxygen." Your body needs oxygen to function and to help it to burn energy. When you breathe you are engaging in aerobic activity because you are taking oxygen into the body. When you train aerobically, by swimming, running, or cycling, for example, you raise your heart rate and increase your body's consumption of oxygen – this not only benefits the heart and lungs and improves circulation, but it also increases the rate at which you burn energy. When you are active your body burns fats and sugars predominantly; but when you are less fit, and as a result have a lower aerobic capacity – or ability to take in and utilize oxygen – your body burns more sugar than fat. As your aerobic capacity increases and you get in better shape, you burn more fat. Even if you are relatively out of shape and just beginning to exercise, you will still burn some fat, and as you become fitter, your body's ability to burn fat will increase.

For your body to burn fat most efficiently, you need to train within your optimum training zone, that is the heart rate in beats per minute at which you burn fat most efficiently (*see chart, at right*). This is generally between 75 and 90 percent of your maximum heart rate (MHR, *see page 17*). If you train above your optimum training zone, you begin to work anaerobically, that is "without oxygen"; you cannot sustain exercise at this rate, and your body will not burn sugar and fat resources in the same way.

Monitor your heart rate while exercising by working for a period of time, then briefly stopping and taking your pulse (*see right and opposite*), for 15 seconds. Multiply that number by four to get your

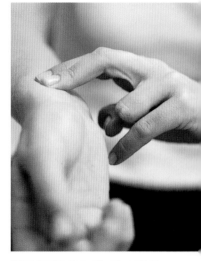

follow the line of your thumb, and use two fingers to feel your pulse on your wrist

heart rate in beats per minute (bpm). The chart below shows the percentage of MHR for different age groups in average bpm. Use the chart to find your optimum training zone.

heart rate chart

age	70% MHR	75% MHR	80% MHR	85% MHR	90% MHR
18–25	139	149	159	169	179
26–30	134	144	153	163	172
31–36	130	140	149	158	168
37–42	126	135	144	153	162
43–50	121	129	138	147	155
50–58	116	124	133	141	149
59–65	110	118	126	134	142
65+	106	114	121	129	136

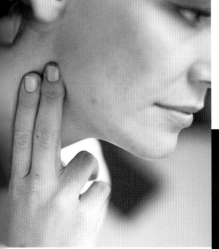

use two fingers to feel your pulse at the side of your neck, below the jawbone

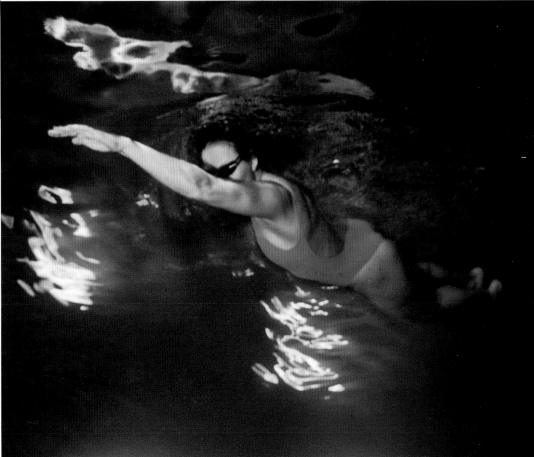

swimming – a great aerobic exercise

the warm-up

Before you begin exercising, prepare your body for the work ahead. Ideally, do five minutes of gentle aerobic exercise such as running or cycling, then perform the stretches below. Use a support such as a railing, wall, or bench to aid balance.

quads

1 ▼ Stand straight with one hand on a support in front of you. Bend one leg back, holding the top of the foot. Keep your knees together. Hold for 8–10 seconds, then repeat for the other leg.

hamstring

2 ▼ Place your heel on a railing or bench in front of you. Bend forward toward your raised foot, keeping your supporting leg slightly bent and your extended leg straight. Bend from the hips rather than curving the back excessively. Hold for 8–10 seconds, then repeat for the other leg.

calves

3 ▼ Lean forward with both hands on a support in front of you. Keep your front leg slightly bent and step back with the other leg, pushing your heel toward the ground. Imagine a straight line running from your shoulder to your back heel. Hold for 8–10 seconds, then repeat for the other leg.

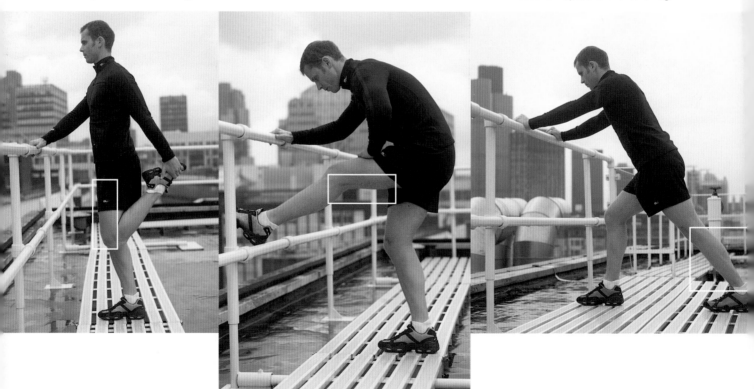

spine

4 ▼ Stand straight with your feet hip-width apart, knees slightly bent. Cross your arms in front of you and raise them to shoulder level. Keep your hips facing forward and rotate your upper body to one side. Hold for 6–8 seconds, then rotate to the other side.

upper back

5 ▼ Stand with your feet hip-width apart, knees slightly bent. Clasp your hands together in front of you and raise your arms to shoulder level. Keeping your elbows slightly bent, stretch into your arms as if pushing something away from you. Hold for 8–10 seconds.

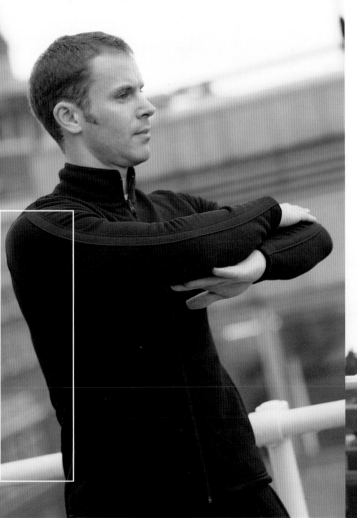

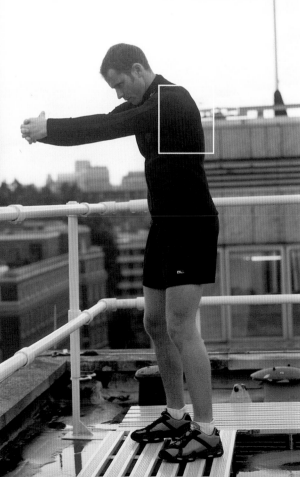

the cooldown

This routine will help to prevent muscle pain after exercise and will create longer, leaner, and more flexible muscles. You can perform all of these exercises on your own, but in many cases, having someone to help you can increase the stretch. Use this time to relax.

hamstrings

1 ▼ Lie on your back with knees bent and feet flat on the floor. Lift one leg, holding it behind the thigh. Gently pull your leg toward you and hold for 8–10 seconds. Bring the leg closer to extend the stretch; repeat for the other leg.

quads

2 ▼ Lie on your front and bend one leg. Reach back with both hands and grasp the front of your foot. Pull your heel toward your buttock, keeping your pelvis on the floor at all times. Hold for 30 seconds, then repeat for the other leg.

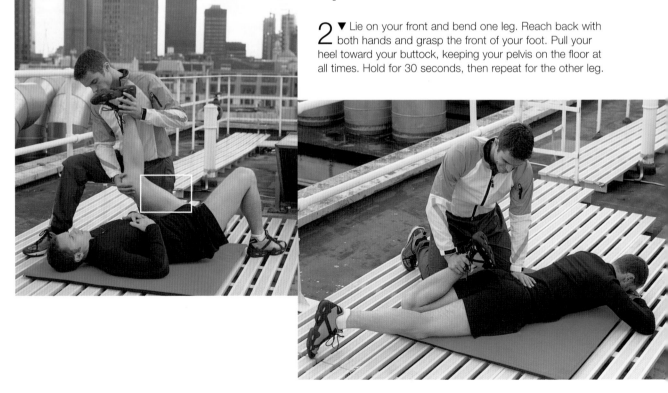

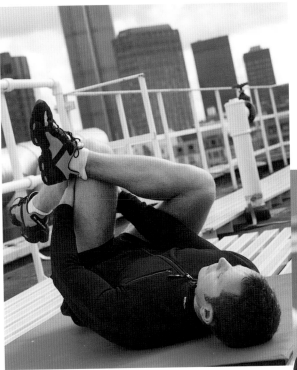

buttocks

3 ◄ Lie on your back with both feet flat on the floor. Cross your right leg over your left, above the knee. Take hold of your left leg behind the thigh and pull both legs toward you until you feel the stretch in your right buttock. Hold for 30 seconds, then cross your legs the other way and stretch the other side.

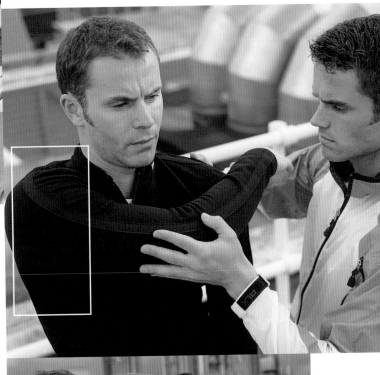

arms

4 ▶ Stand straight with your feet hip-width apart. Raise your right arm to chest level and cross it in front of your body. Place your left hand on your right upper arm and press it firmly into your body until you feel the stretch. Keep your hips facing forward and take care not to twist the upper body. Hold for 10–14 seconds, then repeat for the other arm.

chest

5 ▶ Stand with your feet hip-width apart and knees slightly bent. Clasp your hands behind your back and, keeping your back straight, lift your arms behind you. Lift until you feel the stretch in your chest and in the front of your shoulders. Hold for 10–14 seconds.

running

To get the most out of running, try to look as though you are enjoying it. If you feel comfortable, you are less likely to feel inhibited, and as a result, are more likely to relax. A relaxed posture and good running technique minimize the risk of injury, which, in turn, means that you are more likely to continue running in the future. The more you run, the more you will get out of it and the more you will enjoy it.

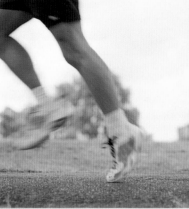

your toes propel you off the ground

running technique

The following tips will reduce your risk of injury and help you to get the most out of running.

• Keep your back flat and your head in line with your spine.

• Hold your stomach muscles tight to maintain good posture.

your arms power you

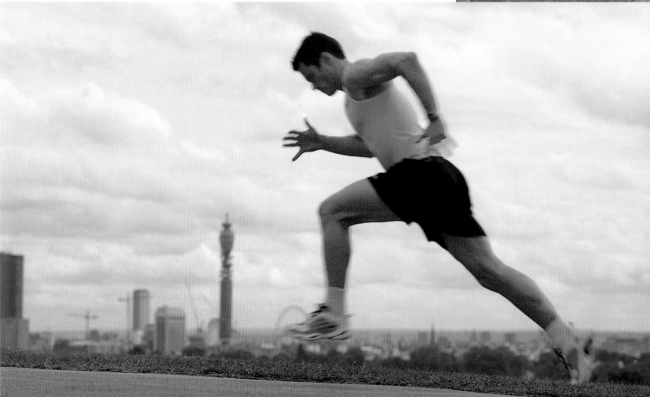

if you feel comfortable running, you will relax   *choose shoes engineered for running*

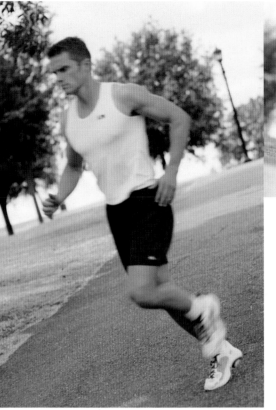

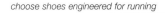

training tips

- Always maintain a heel-toe action when running.

- Always build up the distance and the time that you run in small increments, particularly if you are new to running.

- When you want to quicken your pace, ensure that you work the arms harder as well as the legs.

- When running up hills, alter your body weight forward in the stride to allow for the steeper gradient.

- When sprinting, alter your running action so that you run on the balls of your feet, rather than maintaining the heel-toe action.

- Where possible, run on grass rather than pavement so that there is greater shock absorption for the legs.

- Seek advice from a good sporting goods retailer about the shoes that are most suitable for the way that you run.

- Always wear cotton socks that allow your feet to breathe.

• Create a breathing pattern while running. Aim to breathe in time with your strides. Try to maintain a rate of about three to four strides as you breathe in and three to four strides as you breathe out. You may feel as though you can't keep a long breathing pattern going at first and you may be achieving a two stride pattern, but this will improve with practice.

• Use your arms. They act as a balance for your legs; if you do not use them, your whole body will be thrown out of position. Keep your elbows slightly bent, with all of the movement coming from your shoulder joint.

• Keep your shoulders relaxed; hunched shoulders will impair your arm action and create tension in the neck and shoulders.

• Keep your hands cupped but relaxed. If you are making a tight fist, you are creating tension in your arms as you run.

• Check heel strike. Your heel should strike the ground first, with the sole of your foot rolling through to project you off your toes.

• Watch foot fall. Your foot should land square to the ground, without turning in or out. Landing on the inside or outside of your foot increases the risk of damage to your ankles, knees, and back.

fast walking

swing arms vigorously in time with your strides

Although you walk around every day, it does not necessarily follow that you do it correctly. Fast-paced walking, or power-walking, is a skill in itself and one that, when performed well, can burn many more calories than regular walking.

why fast walk?

Walking makes the ideal cardiovascular work-out when first starting an exercise program because it can be done anywhere and the intensity can be altered by simply speeding up or walking over more hilly terrain. Fast walking makes learning how to work with heart rates very simple since it provides a low-intensity work out so your heart rate is easier to control. Monitoring your heart rate while fast walking can help you to gain a greater understanding of how your body responds to different intensities of exercise. Interval train by walking and then running – beginners should start with a longer walking phase and build up to a longer running phase as they reach a higher level of fitness.

getting the most from fast walking

Correct technique is crucial if you want to get the greatest benefit out of fast walking.

• Check your heel strike. Your heel should strike the ground first, with the sole of your

50

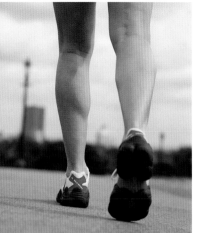

your heel strikes the ground first

foot rolling through to project you off your toes. As you do so, push back hard, using your buttocks and hamstrings (the major muscles at the backs of your legs).

• Keep your body upright, holding your abdominals tight and your lower back firm.

• Use your arms. You can significantly increase the number of calories you burn if you swing your arms rigorously in time with your strides. Bend your elbows at 90° and generate all movement from the shoulder joint. Your arms balance you and prevent you from swinging your hips.

• Hold your shoulders square and don't allow your body to rotate at the waist while walking.

• When you reach a hill, maintain the same posture, keeping your body upright, but allow it to lean forward slightly at the waist. Your legs work harder walking at an angle; take care not to lean too far forward.

• Always maintain a comfortable stride pattern. Keep a natural rhythm, then speed up or down to vary the intensity of your workout.

training tips

The following tips will help you to get the most from fast walking:

• Walk on grass where possible – grass acts as a shock absorber, lessening the impact on the legs.

• Use hills to add greater intensity to your workout.

• Wear the correct footwear; a good sporting goods retailer can advise you on the best walking shoes for your feet.

• If you experience pain in your shins, slow down and avoid steep gradients.

• Keep your abdominals and back firm at all times.

• Use interval training to get the most from your training session.

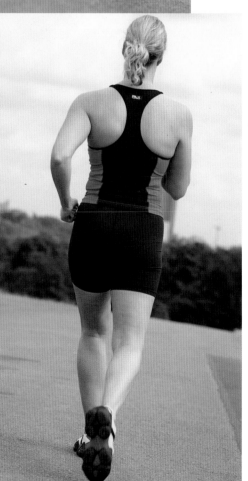

keep your lower back firm

cycling

A great low-impact cardiovascular exercise, cycling works the quadriceps (quads), the muscles at the fronts of the thighs, and tones the legs. Ensure that your bicycle is the correct size for your height and limb length. A good bicycle shop can advise you on this.

cycling technique

Good posture is very important when cycling. Check your body position regularly and make the necessary adjustments to your bicycle to help keep your posture correct. The following points apply whether cycling outdoors or indoors on a cycling machine.

• Adjust the saddle height. At the lowest part of the cyclic action your leg should still be slightly bent. If you have to straighten your leg completely, the saddle is too high and you will put unnecessary strain on the knee joint.

• Keep your back flat to prevent straining the muscles in the middle and lower back.

• Keep the ball and front of your foot placed firmly on the pedals. As you cycle, the force of the movement is generated by the quads, then transferred through the ball of the foot.

using the cycling machine

Cycling on a stationary bicycle may seem straightforward, but good technique is just as important, and the better it is, the more effective your workout will be.

• Choose an appropriate speed in relation to the resistance – 85 to 90 revolutions per minute (rpm) is the optimum level for fat

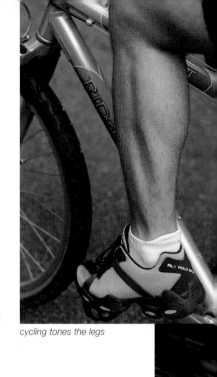

cycling tones the legs

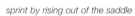

sprint by rising out of the saddle

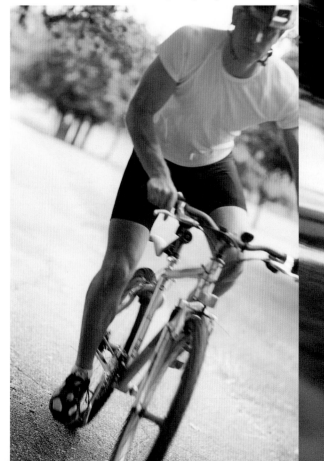

burning. Work hard enough to test your legs, heart, and lungs. Freewheeling will not provide an effective workout, nor will a high resistance level that means you can hardly pedal at all.

• Try a spinning class to add variety to your cycling routine.

• Work each leg in turn – put more pressure on one leg, then alternate and cycle harder with the other leg.

even better with fresh air

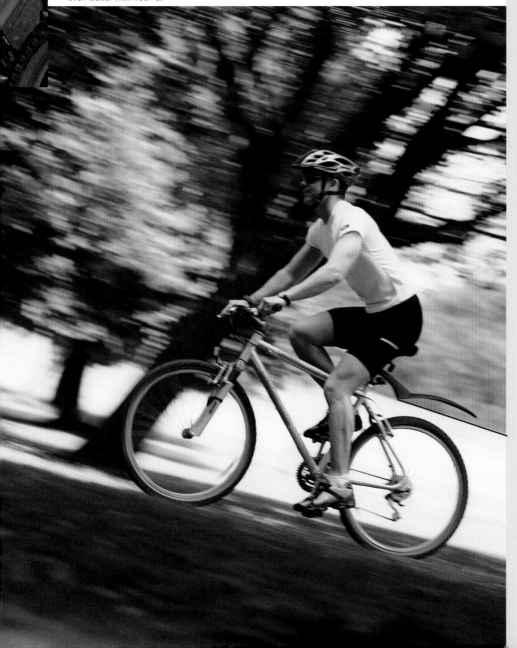

training tips

The following tips will help you to get the most benefit from your cycling sessions:

● Interval train. Choose a moderate resistance that allows you to work in your optimum training zone (*see page 43*), then raise the intensity by increasing the resistance, rising out of the saddle, and sprinting for short periods.

● When cycling outdoors, plan routes that will involve cycling over hills as this will vary the intensity of your workout.

● Maintain good posture at all times, especially when fatigued – there may be a tendency to hunch over the handle bars when tired.

● If you cycle for long periods, wear padded cycling shorts that help to cushion your groin against the saddle.

swimming

One of the most popular sports in the US, swimming builds strength and tones the body; it can also be a fantastic low-impact cardiovascular workout. Get the most out of it by really working hard – this will not only bring greater health benefits, it will also reduce the monotony factor that swimming can sometimes induce.

getting the most from swimming

A gentle 30-minute swim has its benefits, but for a good aerobic workout, really push yourself, working your heart and lungs to near maximum capacity as much as possible (*see panel*).

front crawl technique

The most common problem that people have with the front crawl is breathing. Remember to relax when practicing new technique, and keep the stroke as long as possible.

• Breathe properly: breathe out through your mouth while your head is in the water, and turn your head to one side, so your ear is by your shoulder, when you breathe in. Practice with one arm on a kick board and the other pulling – breathe on the same side as the arm that is pulling.

• Position your arms correctly: reach directly in front of you so your hand enters the water in line with your shoulder (*see right*).

• Reach directly in front of you and pull your hand through the center line of your body as

front crawl – pull through the center line of your body

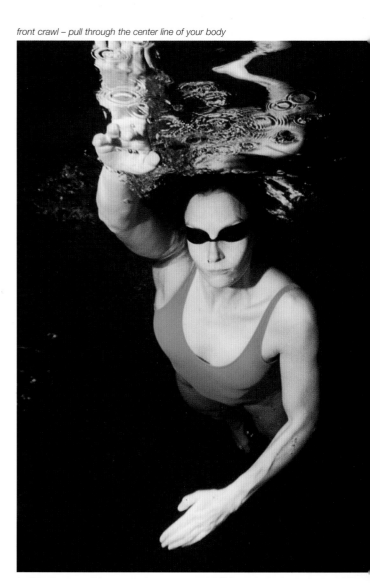

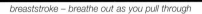

breaststroke – breathe out as you pull through

The following tips will help you to get more out of swimming, but aim to improve your fitness levels and technique as well:

• Stretch before you enter the water. Follow a basic warm-up routine (*see pages 44–5*).

• Warm up in the water. Before you begin the session in earnest, swim two or three slower lengths, varying your strokes.

• Interval train. Instead of swimming up and down at the same speed, vary your pace. For example, swim one length very fast, then swim two lengths at a more leisurely pace.

• Alternate strokes. Swim one length of a stroke you find more difficult, then swim two lengths of a stroke that you find easier.

• Improve technique and strength by practicing with flotation boards.

• Cool down at the end of the session. Do two lengths at a comfortable pace, then dry off and follow a basic cool-down routine (*see pages 46–7*).

you execute each stroke. Keep a slight bend in the elbow.
• Cup your hands as you pull through the stroke.
• Kick from the hips, not from the knees.
• Keep your feet pointed, but relaxed.

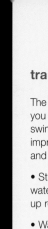

breaststroke – glide between strokes

breaststroke technique

Correct technique is important. It will improve your workout times and reduce the risk of muscle injury, but it will also increase your enjoyment of swimming.

• Breathe properly: place your head in the water when your arms are extended forward, and breathe out through your mouth or nose. As you pull your arms around and then together, bring your head out of the water and breathe in through your mouth.
• Don't kick too wide.
• Don't pull your arms out too wide; keep the stroke quite narrow.
• Turn your feet out as you kick back; the soles of your feet should face the back wall of the pool. This helps to propel you through the water.
• Keep your movements smooth and rhythmic. You should glide forward between strokes without having to work.

rowing

This is an excellent aerobic exercise that works the upper and lower body at the same time. However, since rowing is a more technical discipline that requires some coordination, it is easy to perform it incorrectly and, as a result, not get the maximum benefit from it.

using the rowing machine

The start of the rowing stroke is called the "catch" position. Your legs should be bent, with the knees tucked in close to the chest. Your arms should be straight, extended directly in front of you at shoulder level, and you should have a firm grip on the handles, with your hands positioned directly above your toes. Your torso should tilt forward slightly while your back is held firm.

Start the first stroke by straightening your legs, using your leg muscles to power the movement and keeping your arms extended in front of you. Keep your torso in the catch position

your legs power the stroke as you pull back

the start, or "catch," position

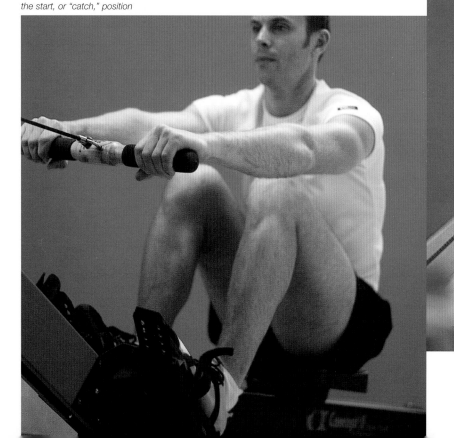

as you start to pull back. Keep your arms straight until they reach the knees, then lean back slightly, pulling the handle toward your chest. Pull your shoulders back so your elbows bend just behind your body. Your legs should be straight and your body tilted back slightly. As you return to the start position, stretch your arms forward and straighten them as you tilt the body forward, pivoting off the hips. As you slide forward, bend your legs and tuck your knees up close to your chest. Take care not to "lock" your legs straight since this can put unnecessary strain on the knees – they should stay slightly bent. Your arms should be straight in the finish position, and your body should tilt forward slightly.

hold the back firm

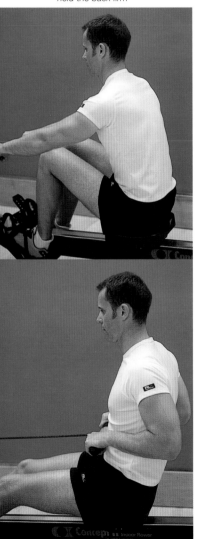

legs are slightly bent at finish

key points for good technique

To get the most out of your session, remember the following points.

• Generate the bulk of the stroke power from the legs. If your arms tire before your legs, you need to check and correct your technique.

• Avoid putting excessive strain on the back. Although the technique demands a slight pivoting action from the lower back, use the legs and not the back to generate power. Take care not to lean too far back at the end of the stroke.

• Keep your stroke rate at about 25–35 strokes per minute (spm). Don't go for speed at the expense of technique.

• Work at a heart rate that is 10 beats per minute (bpm, *see pages 42–3*) slower than for other aerobic activities, such as cycling or running.

training tips

Try these training tips to help you get the most out of your rowing session:

● Keep your grip on the handle or "oar" relaxed, otherwise your forearms will tire prematurely.

● Exhale with the effort, as you pull back, and inhale as you return to the start position.

● If you wear loose clothing such as a t-shirt, tuck it in, otherwise it may get caught in the sliding seat.

● Record your best 500 m time, then keep retesting yourself and work toward beating it.

● Interval train for a time-efficient, high-calorie-burning workout. Work at a high intensity, ease off slightly and recover, then work at high intensity again.

resistance training

The goal of my program is not only to help you to feel healthier and improve your fitness level; it is also to help you to lose excess body fat. A specially tailored resistance training program can enable you to achieve that goal.

intensity theory

Each phase in the program takes you through a sequence of exercises, each of which needs to be repeated a given number of times to ensure its effectiveness. Depending on the exercise, you may also need to lift weights. Each exercise is accompanied by a chart that tells you how many repetitions you need to perform. Do the number of repetitions specified and no more. If the chart gives a number of repetitions maximum, or RM, you need to choose a weight that will allow you to do that number of repetitions and no more. You will need to experiment to find the correct weight – you should feel that by the last two or three repetitions you are reaching your maximum and are just able to finish the set.

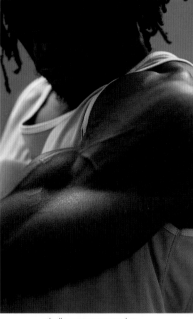
challenge your muscles

The number of repetitions for each exercise tests your body to the point where you increase overall muscle utilization, but without gaining muscle mass. Doing fewer repetitions with a higher weight is more likely to build muscle mass. Doing a greater number of repetitions with a lower weight will build muscle endurance rather than bulk. However, our bodies do respond to different forms of training, and it is possible to include high weight/low repetition sets in a program without building muscle mass. The important thing is to challenge your muscles by varying your weights, repetitions, and speed. My resistance training program sets the best foundations for fitness; if you work through each of the phases, you can achieve results that will stay with you long after you have completed the program.

white and red muscle fibers

Muscles are made up of white fast-twitch fibers and red slow-twitch fibers. The different muscle fibers work in different ways, depending on how they are tested. Not everyone has the same ratio of white to red muscle fibers. A sprinter has more white fibers and will probably have a more muscular, bulky physique than a marathon runner who, with many more red fibers, will have a slighter build.

Consider your own body type. If you are stronger and find it easy to build muscle, your body will probably respond better to aerobic and endurance exercise and you should keep your heavy weight work to a minimum. If you are a slighter build, you are probably more suited to interval training and can use heavier weights. Because my program combines aerobic and resistance training, it is suitable for all body types; but you can still use this information to make minor adjustments to the way you train once you have finished the program. Unfortunately, because we all have different body types, the exercise you want to do may not always be the one most suitable for you. Variety is the key to testing all your muscle fibers effectively.

aim for lasting results

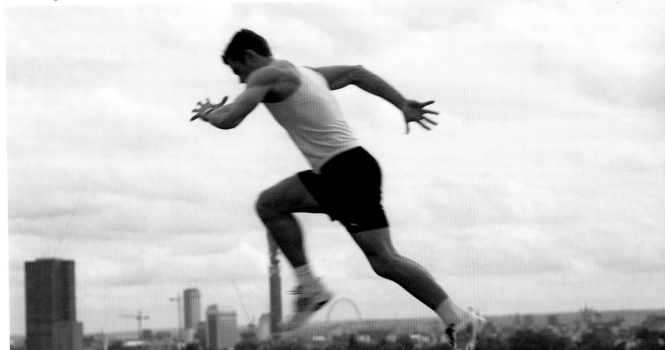

weight training

People often fear that working with weights will build bulky muscles. This is not true. In fact, weight training is essential for shaping and toning the body.

fat reduction and water retention in muscles

Your body is made up of between 60 and 65 percent water. Sixty-two percent of it is stored in the body intracellularly, or within the cells; the remaining 38 percent is stored extracellularly, or outside of the cells, in blood plasma, saliva, spinal fluid, and fluid secreted by glands, for example.

When you exercise aerobically, your body secretes large amounts of fluid as sweat – drinking water after aerobic exercise replenishes your body's fluid levels. With resistance training, people are less inclined to drink water because they don't lose as much fluid in the obvious way, through sweating. However, because a large amount of fluid is stored within the muscles, and in fact a process of acidic buildup begins as a result of resistance training, it is just as important to drink water during and after weight training. It ensures a healthy transfer of water between all of your body's tissues and prevents water retention since your body does not feel that it needs to hold on to water for emergencies.

A low-calorie diet will achieve weight loss, but the weight will consist of 70 percent water (lost mostly from the muscles, which are made up of 75 percent water), 25 percent fat, and five percent proteins. Weight training combined with a sensible eating plan, as outlined in the program, ensures that the muscles are hydrated enough intracellularly so that they function efficiently, and that weight loss is achieved through fat reduction and not fluid loss. Your metabolic rate will also rise, which will mean that you lose excess fat and are less likely to retain water.

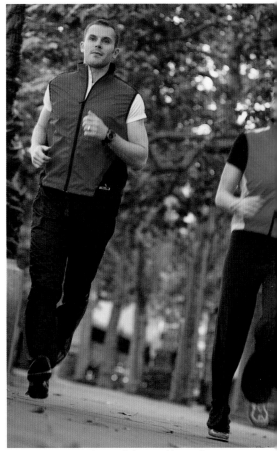

you sweat more during aerobic exercise

reversibility

"If you don't use it, you lose it." In fact, I would alter this to "If you don't keep testing it, you lose it." Your body is an efficient machine, but it is also rather cunning. As it gets used to an exercise, it adapts so that it can perform it with less effort. If you ran the same route at the same pace every day, your body would gradually begin to put less effort into it. Eventually, you would reach a point where you would plateau – you might run for the same time, but you would not be getting fitter.

Challenge yourself; don't fall into the "comfort zone." Push yourself constantly and vary your exercises and routines. If the exercises stay the same, change the order in which you do them and vary the intensity. If you run, take a different route; do a set of heavy weights when you might normally have done a set of light ones. The program introduces change, but be aware of the body's tendency toward complacency. The downside may be that you will never reach a point where you find the exercise easy, but then you wouldn't be pushing yourself as hard as you could be.

vary your training routine

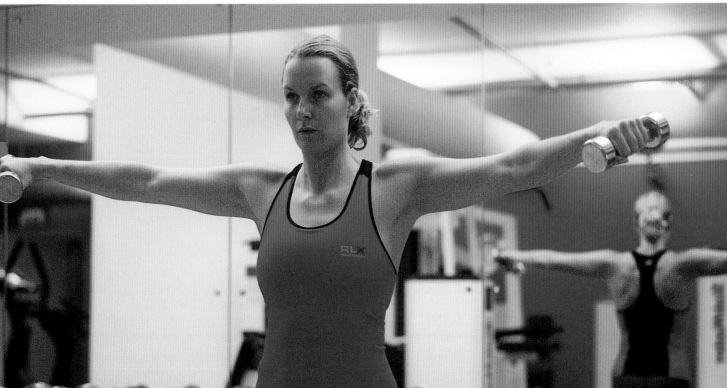

flexibility

Increased muscle flexibility makes the physical demands of daily life easier, but it will also help prevent postural problems that can cause discomfort in the back, shoulders, and neck.

good flexibility

There is more to good flexibility than simply being able to bend over and touch your toes. It should mean that you can perform a wide range of movement, enjoy good mobility, and maintain good posture at all times.

If you intend to take up a new sport or get involved in an activity that will put different physical demands on your body, ensure that you are flexible enough before you begin. Don't expect the sport or activity to give you the flexibility. You will simply increase the likelihood of injuring yourself or straining a muscle. Prior to exercise, prepare you muscles by gently stretching them. If the activity will involve a new range of movement, try to gently stretch the muscles that will be used. There is no need to stretch excessively – this won't increase your flexibility. As the muscle elongates, relax into the stretch. Try to spend between five and 10 minutes a day doing a general stretching routine (*see pages 44–7*). The older you get, the more important it becomes to maintain flexibility. Spend time now improving your mobility and you will spend less time later wishing that you had done it before.

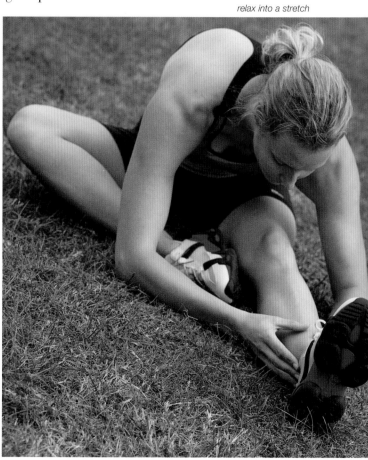

relax into a stretch

correct posture

If you have ever looked at a photograph of yourself that was taken without you realizing, you may have been surprised by your posture.

Unposed pictures can reveal how you actually hold yourself, and sometimes it can come as quite a shock.

The most common postural problem occurs when the head and shoulders "roll" forward, causing a stooped look. Often this is the result of long hours spent hunched over a desk. The muscles in the chest and at the front of the shoulders tighten and, combined with a weak upper back, this can cause the back and neck to arch. This not only increases your risk of spine injury, but it also has the effect of making you look older and shorter.

If you find that your butt is not as pert as it once was, it may be that your pelvis has shifted position. A "tilted" pelvis, which tucks under at the base of the spine, can give your butt an undesirable "saggy" appearance. The lengthening effect this has on your spine can make your legs look shorter and produce an undesirable "pot-bellied" effect, but it may also cause back pain.

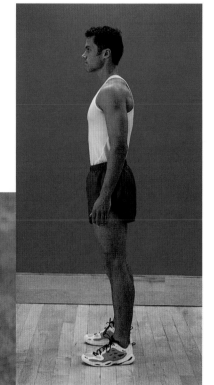

assess your posture

Your knees, and the strength of the muscles around them, can also affect your posture. Stand facing a mirror and assess the comparative size and shape of your knees. Perform a shallow knee bend and look at whether your knees bend forward in line with your ankles and hips. You should be able to draw two imaginary lines down from your hips to your knees to your middle toe. If, while bending, your knees sway either inside or outside that line, there may be some knee joint misalignment. This can be due to muscle over- or underdevelopment, which give a "knock-kneed" or "bow-legged" appearance to the legs, but can also be a major cause of hip and back problems. You can counteract such problems by increasing the strength and flexibility of all the muscles of the legs and lower back.

Many people who are unhappy with their body shape attribute it to excess body fat when in fact it is just as likely to be related to poor posture. Assess your posture and you may find the key to attaining the body you desire.

back problems

In the past decade there has been a five-fold increase in the number of working days lost through people suffering from back problems. Back pain is one of the most common complaints, yet in the majority of cases it can be prevented.

common causes

In some cases, back pain may be unavoidable. It can be caused by a genetic postural abnormality or it may be the result of excessive strain. However, many people suffer needlessly from back pain. It can occur when one or more of the muscles that support the spine tighten and either push or pull the spine out of position. The muscles that most commonly cause this are the hamstrings, which are situated at the backs of the thighs, and the hip flexor, which is attached to the pelvis. When the hamstrings are very tight, they limit mobility around the hip and knees, and the body compensates for this by repositioning itself so the pelvis tilts further forward. Because the hip flexor is attached to the pelvic area, it can pull the pelvis. Too much time spent sitting down can allow the hamstrings and hip flexor to shorten and become stiff, which alters your posture and, ultimately, causes back pain.

Weak abdominals and a weak lower back can also contribute to back problems. Your upper and lower body put pressure on the trunk area to rotate, bend, and extend, so it must be strong as it acts as a "pivot" point for this movement. Although your spine can withstand enormous pressure from a single direction, constant strain from a number of directions can cause back pain and irreparable damage.

Ensure that you stretch, before and after exercise, by following the suggested warm-up and cooldown routines *(see pages 44–7)*, and make sure that you include abdominal and lower back exercises in your regular exercise routine, since they will help protect your back from injury.

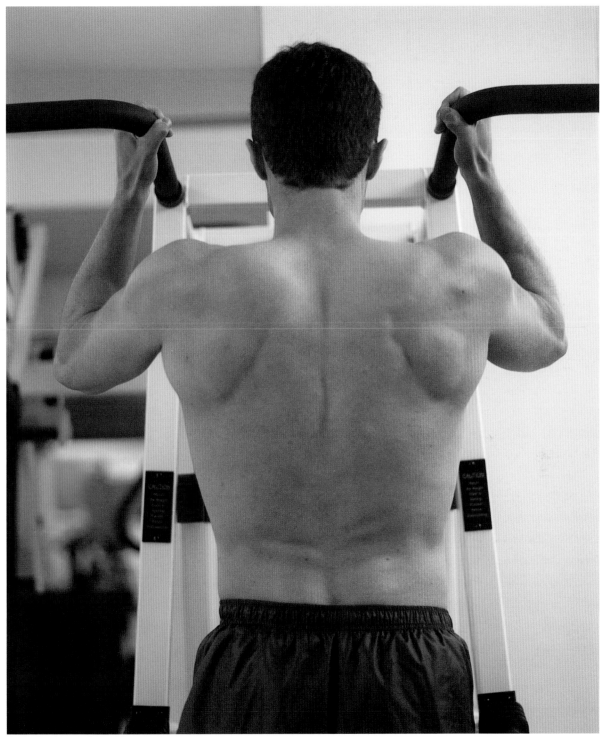

the trunk acts as a pivot point

neck problems

Many people suffer from pain and stiffness in the neck and shoulders as a result of poor posture, stress, and general tension. Often this can cause discomfort in other parts of the body.

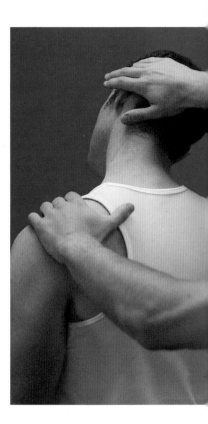

the causes

When faced with a situation that we find stressful, the body's instinctive reaction is to produce adrenaline to prepare it to either confront the danger or to run away from it – the fight or flight mechanism. These days, this type of physical response to stress is inappropriate. We tend to internalize stress and it manifests itself as tension, which may be concentrated in various parts of the body. More often than not, we experience it quite literally as a "pain in the neck." Stiffness and pain in the neck and shoulder muscles can also cause headaches, but there are steps you can take to ease any discomfort.

looking after your neck and shoulders

The most effective way to reduce tension in the neck and shoulders is either to apply heat to the area or to use massage, which promotes blood flow. Try applying a warm hot water bottle to the affected area, or concentrating gentle pressure on it by aiming comfortably hot water from a shower head at it (incidentally, this technique has proven to be very effective in the treatment of mild insomnia).

Alternatively, try massaging the neck and shoulder area – you don't necessarily need a therapist to do this for you, but it will make the experience far more enjoyable. Start at the outside of the shoulder, reaching across with the opposite hand. Work inward using a circular motion, pressing gently into the muscles of the shoulder and neck to promote blood flow. Combining gentle massage and heat treatment will provide effective relief from muscle strain and need take only 10–15 minutes a few times a week.

foot problems

tension can be a pain in the neck

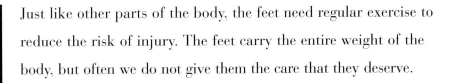

Just like other parts of the body, the feet need regular exercise to reduce the risk of injury. The feet carry the entire weight of the body, but often we do not give them the care that they deserve.

heel and arch problems

Our weight is fairly evenly distributed when we walk, but when we run, each heel hits the ground with great force and with the weight of the whole body behind it. Running increases the risk of injury, but you can protect your feet by looking after them and wearing good shoes.

The delicate arch area of the foot can be affected by our shoes and by the way that we walk. People walk in different ways, and the foot adapts accordingly. Some walk with their weight concentrated on the outside of the feet, or supinate, while others walk with their weight concentrated on the inside of the feet, or pronate. There are flat-footed people, but there are also people who walk perfectly. The soles of a well-worn pair of shoes hold the clues to the way that you walk.

old shoes hold the clues

caring for your feet

Exercise your feet: strengthen the arch area by standing and tensing your feet as if trying to grip the floor. Whenever possible, walk around without shoes. Shoes support the arch rather than the muscles in the feet having to do so, which allows the muscles to become weak. This can result in an increased risk of injury as well as tendon damage and fallen arches. Choose your shoes with care – they should be suitable for the sport that you use them for, but also for the way that you walk and run. The most expensive shoes are not necessarily the best.

nutrition

The word "diet" does not have to induce feelings of panic. The diet guidelines in my program are not intended to achieve instant weight loss, but they will introduce you to a new and more wholesome way of eating that will nourish your body.

what is a diet?

The dictionary definition of a diet is "the nutritional outline of what a person consumes." With the number of fad diets and miracle weight loss plans that have been published over the years, our perception of what a diet is has changed considerably.

We now equate a diet with a strategy for achieving weight loss – the more dramatic the better and in as short a time period as possible. Most of us know that this is a very unhealthy approach to eating that will only put unnecessary strain on the body. Diets that insist that you must count calories, eat less fat, eat more fat, weigh food, or eliminate certain foods from your diet altogether, help to turn food into an enemy when it is really there to nourish you and to be enjoyed. I once heard a saying: "The quicker the weight comes off, the quicker it goes back on," and unfortunately this is too often true of fad diets that promise a lot.

If you are taken in by fad diets that make big promises, you will inevitably become locked into a cycle of yo-yo dieting (*see page 26*). Clients who swore by that miracle diet that helped them to lose weight years ago now fight a constant battle to keep their weight down.

A diet should fit into your lifestyle. It should encourage you to eat a range of different foods and should be enjoyable, so that you can carry on with it for the rest of your life.

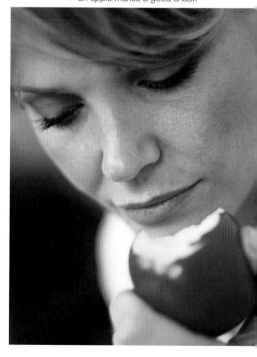
an apple makes a good snack

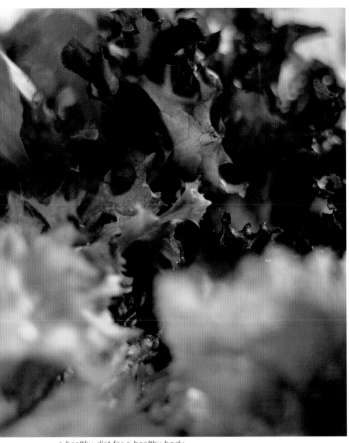

a healthy diet for a healthy body

a healthy diet

Our diet should provide us with all of the nutrients we need to maintain a healthy body. It should be low in processed foods and foods that include preservatives and artificial additives. A healthy diet helps to maintain a healthy body: it fuels energy levels and helps us to fight stress, protect against illness, and maintain a body shape that we are happy with. It gives the body what it needs, when it needs it, so you don't feel inclined to starve yourself or overeat.

Feeling tired and bloated after eating is normal for many people, but this usually means you have overeaten and your body is having trouble digesting food. After a meal you should feel satisfied and pleasantly full. A good diet, as outlined in the program, provides the body with a constant supply of energy throughout the day. You should start the day with a wholesome breakfast of easily digestible food (*see pages 74–5*). Lunch should be in the middle of the day, when you need the most energy, and should consist of complex carbohydrates that will fuel the body through the afternoon (*see pages 90–1*). Your evening meal should be light and easy to digest because you need less energy in the evening when you are resting (*see pages 104–5*). Light snacks that are low in sugar and fat can help to sustain you between meals; snacks high in sugar and fat will only lock you into a cycle of craving where you suffer energy highs and lows and inevitably eat more (*see pages 114–15*).

Most importantly, a good diet should allow you to enjoy food rather than fear it. Aim to follow the program's nutritional guidelines about 80 percent of the time, and treat yourself to foods that you enjoy but which are not in the program the other 20 percent of the time.

acid and alkaline food

The acid/alkaline balance in the body is important. It is better to eat a more alkaline diet because high acid levels can upset the healthy functioning of the body. Generally, people tend to eat a more acidic diet, but acid levels can also build up in the body as a result of stress, disease, inactivity, and poor diet. The nutritional goals outlined in the program encourage you to eat more alkaline-forming foods since they will help to combat acid buildup. Listed on these two pages are a variety of mostly familiar foods and an indication of whether they are acid or alkaline forming in the body. (Some foods are shown as neutral, since they are neither acid nor alkaline.)

vegetables

Asparagus (very alkaline)

Brussels sprouts (alkaline)

Broccoli (alkaline)

Cabbage (alkaline)

Cauliflower (alkaline)

Leeks (alkaline)

Mushrooms (neutral)

Onion (alkaline)

Parsnips (alkaline)

Peppers (alkaline)

Potatoes (alkaline)

Rhubarb (alkaline)

Spinach (alkaline)

Sweet corn (alkaline)

Tomatoes (acid)

Watercress (very alkaline)

fruit

Apples (alkaline)

Bananas (alkaline)

Berries (alkaline)

Grapes (alkaline)

Lemons (alkaline)

Mangoes (very alkaline)

Melon (very alkaline)

Oranges (neutral)

Pears (alkaline)

Plums (acid)

Strawberries (alkaline)

carbohydrates

Pasta

Wholegrain with artichoke flour (alkaline)

Wholemeal (neutral)

White (acid)

Potatoes (alkaline if eaten with skin, acid if eaten without skin)

Popcorn

Plain (neutral)

With butter (acid)

With salt (acid)

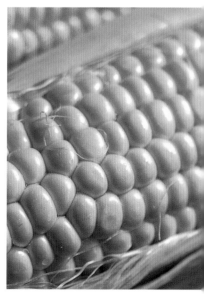

sweet corn is alkaline forming

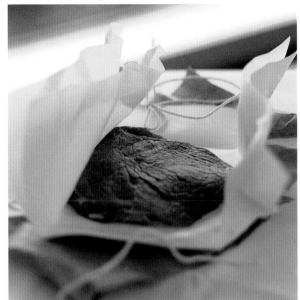
beef is very acid forming

grains

Amaranth (alkaline)

Bleached wheat (acid)

Buckwheat (acid)

Couscous (neutral)

Millet (alkaline)

Oats (neutral)

Quinoa (alkaline)

Rye (acid)

White rice (acid)

Whole wheat (alkaline)

Wild rice (alkaline)

beans and pulses

Adzuki beans (neutral)

Green beans (alkaline)

Kidney beans (neutral)

Lentils (alkaline)

Mung beans (neutral)

Peas (alkaline)

Pinto beans (neutral)

Soybeans (alkaline)

String beans (alkaline)

nuts

Almonds (alkaline)

Brazil (neutral)

Cashews (acid)

Chestnuts (alkaline)

Coconut (alkaline)

Pecans (neutral)

Pistachio (neutral)

Walnuts (neutral)

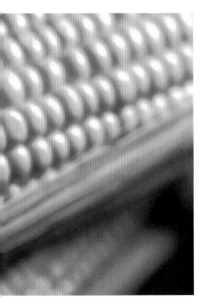

seeds

Pumpkin (neutral)

Sesame (alkaline)

Sunflower (neutral)

Wheatgerm (acid)

meat and fish

Beef (very acid)

Chicken (acid)

Lamb (very acid)

Oily fish (neutral)

Other fish (acid)

Pork (very acid)

Turkey (acid)

animal products

Cheese (acid)

Cow's milk (acid)

Cream (neutral)

Goat's milk (neutral)

Plain yogurt (neutral)

Sweetened yogurt (acid)

oils and fats

Almond oil (neutral)

Animal fats (acid)

Avocado (neutral)

Butter (neutral)

Margarine (neutral)

Olive (alkaline)

Sesame (neutral)

71

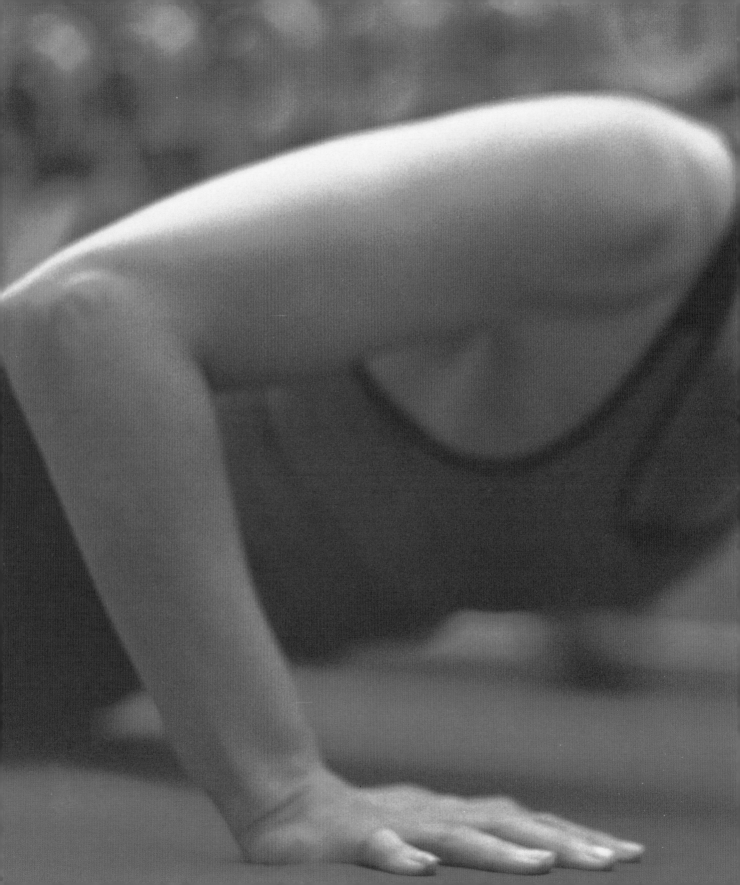

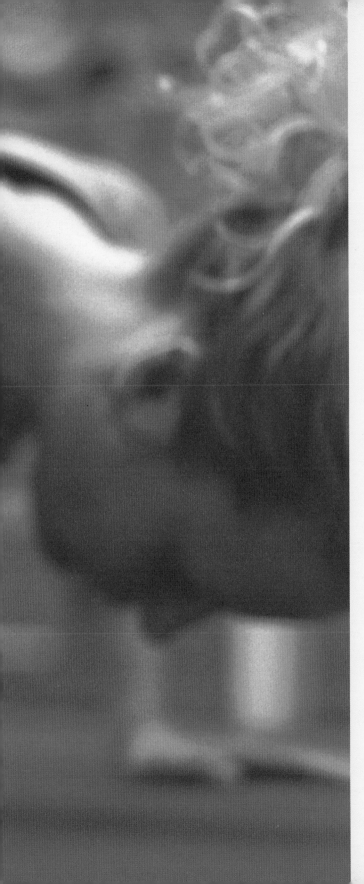

phase one

forming

The aim of Phase One is to condition and prepare

a base

the body, laying the foundations of good fitness

of fitness

that will enable you to rise to the challenges ahead.

Achieving the nutritional goals will help to

energize your body. Spend 21 days on this phase

of the program.

nutritional goals

With a few simple changes to your diet, you begin detoxification and boost your energy levels as a result. Keep your goals in mind: this is where you set the foundations for the work that lies ahead.

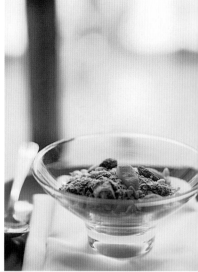

make your own wheat-free muesli

breakfast goals
• Try to eat breakfast every day

phase 1 goals
• Drink at least 3 pints (1.5 liters) of water every day
• Eat four pieces of fruit every day
• Eat at least three portions of fresh vegetables every day

If you scored as highly acidic in the Nutritional Questionnaire *(see pages 32–3)*, **add the following goals:**
• Remove nearly all red meat from your diet; allow it as part of one meal a week
• Increase your water intake from 3 pints (1.5 liters) to 4 pints (2 liters) per day
• Cut wheat products such as bread, pasta, couscous, and cereals from at least one of your daily meals

water
Drinking more water enables the body to function more efficiently and can even help shed weight since it enables the body to flush out retained fluids. The 3–4 pints (1.5–2 liters) of liquid that you need to drink every day should be almost exclusively water, although you can include herbal tea and diluted unsweetened fruit juices. Tea, coffee, sweetened juices from concentrate, carbonated drinks, and alcohol do not count as water.

fresh fruit and vegetables
Packed with vitamins and minerals and essential to the healthy functioning of the body, fresh fruit and vegetables are easy to digest and energize and detoxify the body as well as boosting the immune system. Remember not to cook the goodness out of fresh produce, and to buy organic whenever possible.

breakfast

A healthy breakfast kick-starts the metabolism. Try to include wholesome, nutrient-rich, easily digestible foods (*see panel*) since they will boost your energy levels and help to fuel your body for the rest of the day. Avoid eating cooked food for breakfast (except oatmeal) and, whenever possible, go for foods in their uncooked, raw state – cooking tends to either add fat or destroy nutrients. Try to avoid wheat (*see pages 70–1*) and don't become reliant on toast or breakfast cereal, although they are fine a couple of times a week. If you buy breakfast cereal, choose a variety that is low in sugar and salt, and preferably organic.

Most important of all, vary your options. If you eat the same breakfast cereal every day, the body is not challenged and cannot absorb nutrients from it in the same way. Smoothies (*see panel*) are a healthy breakfast option: simply blend the ingredients to make a drinkable consistency.

smoothies are quick and nutritious

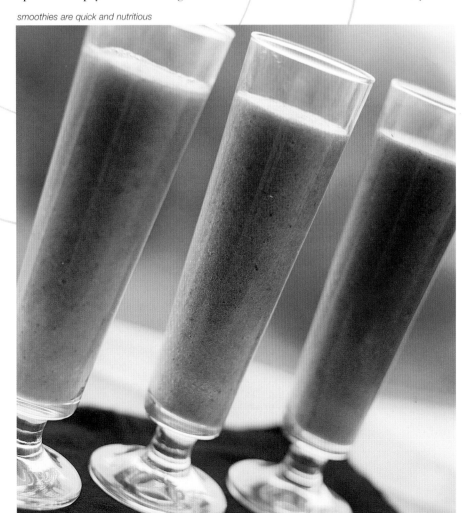

healthy breakfasts

Wheat-free muesli Use organic rolled oats for half the mixture and add natural unsweetened puffed rice, sesame seeds, almonds, sunflower seeds, linseeds, dried apricots, raisins, and dried banana to make up the other half.

Fresh fruit Try melons, strawberries, bananas, blueberries, kiwis, and peaches; eat fewer oranges and grapefruits since they are more acidic. Add yogurt, if preferred, but no more than twice a week.

A detox smoothie Blend fresh melon, kiwi, pineapple juice, and ice.

An energizing smoothie Blend fresh pear, apple, kiwi, carrot juice, and ice.

The perfect breakfast smoothie Blend fresh strawberries, banana, pineapple juice, orange juice, a little low-fat plain yogurt, and ice.

Wholemeal toast Spread with a little butter (not margarine) and honey or jam. Aim to eat butter no more than twice a week.

Oatmeal Make with organic rolled oats, if possible.

aerobic training

The aim of the aerobic training in Phase One is to strengthen your heart and lungs and build a healthy cardiovascular system. You work at a constant heart rate for the whole of your workout, which will build endurance and prepare your body for the work ahead.

An aerobic training program has three elements: frequency, which is how often you exercise; intensity, which is how hard you exercise – you should always work within your optimum training zone (*see page 43*), which is between 75 and 90 percent of your MHR (*see page 17*); and time, which is the duration of your exercise session. Each of these elements will vary depending on your fitness level (*see chart, below*) and phase in the program.

    Begin by doing five minutes of gentle aerobic exercise, such as jogging or cycling, then follow the warm-up routine (*see pages 44–5*). Start your aerobic exercise, taking your heart rate to the correct intensity in the heart rate chart (*see page 43*). Monitor your heart rate while exercising by working for a period of time, then stopping briefly and taking your pulse (*see pages 42–3*), or by using a heart rate monitor. At this stage be aware of how you feel at different heart rates. You will soon find that you can recognize what heart rate you are working at by how you feel, and measuring heart rate will not be as necessary.

phase 1 endurance development constant heart rate training chart

level	◡	◡◡	◡◡◡
frequency	3 per week	4 per week	5 per week
intensity	70% MHR	75% MHR	80% MHR
time	25 mins	23-35 mins	45-60 mins

If, when you begin, you find it difficult to exercise for the specified time for your fitness level, gradually build up to it. Remember, you can vary your exercises as long as you work for the total time shown. You could do three different exercises in the time – cycling, walking, and rowing, for example – if you preferred.

resistance training

Here, you work the major muscles and build strength. Follow two of your weekly aerobic training sessions with the resistance training program below. Once you are familiar with the exercises (*see pages 78–87*), photocopy this page and refer to it in the gym.

phase 1 resistance training chart

level			
leg extensions	15 rm	12 rm	10 rm
leg curls	15 rm	15 rm	15 rm
squats	25 rm	15 rm	15 rm
lunges	25 rm	25 rm	20 rm
perform	2 sets	3 sets	4 sets
push-ups	15	20	30
lat pull-downs	15 rm	15 rm	-
pull-ups	-	-	10
bicep curls	20 rm	20 rm	15 rm
hammer curls	20 rm	20 rm	15 rm
tricep extensions/ overheads	20 rm	20 rm	15 rm
perform	2 sets	3 sets	4 sets
chest press	20 rm	20 rm	15 rm
single arm row	18 rm	18 rm	15 rm
pec flys	15 rm	15 rm	10 rm
perform	2 sets	3 sets	4 sets

The resistance training programs use repetition maximums (rm) to work out the correct weight with which to train (*see page 58*). The lower the rm, the heavier the weight you need to lift to reach fatigue in the reps suggested. The last three reps should always feel difficult – if this is not the case, it means that you are not using enough weight. Experiment – if you are unable to complete the suggested number of reps, your weights are too heavy and you should lower weight. As you get stronger, make sure that you increase your weights so that you continue to see improvements and still find the last three reps of any set difficult.

Complete the required number of sets for each sequence of exercises in the chart before you move on to the next sequence of exercises – do the required number of sets until you finish the program.

resistance exercises

Phase One resistance training aims to develop and tone the major muscles of the body. This will increase the body's metabolic rate and help it to burn fat more efficiently. The exercises are divided into sequences. Do the number of sets specified for your fitness level (*see page 77*).

---

leg extensions

This exercise works the quadriceps, or quads, the powerful muscles at the fronts of the thighs. Take three seconds to lift, then three seconds to return to the start position.

1 ▶ Sit with your ankles hooked behind the roller pad and your legs positioned at 90°. Keep your toes pointing forward to ensure that you work all muscles in the area evenly. Pointing the toes to one side can distort leg shape. Hold the handles at the side of the machine to prevent straining the lower back.

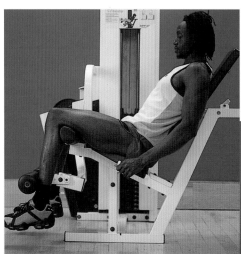

2 ▼ Slowly extend your legs until they are straight. Hold for about half a second, then slowly return to the start position, but don't allow the weights to "touch down." Remember to exhale as you lift the weights and inhale as you lower them.

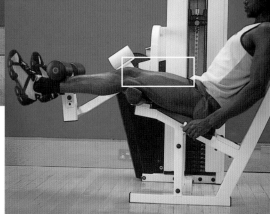

level	◠	◠◠	◠◠◠
repetitions	15 rm	12 rm	10 rm

leg curls

The hamstrings are the large muscles at the backs of the thighs. Hamstring work can reward you with longer-looking legs and a slimmer butt. As the muscles develop, they can also increase your body's calorie-burning potential.

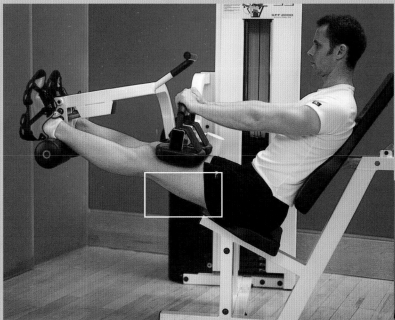

1 ◄ Sit with your legs extended and your ankles on top of the roller pad. Your back should be at right angles to your legs, and your lower back should be supported throughout the exercise. Aim to spread the movement over 6 seconds: 3 seconds to bend the legs and 3 seconds to extend them.

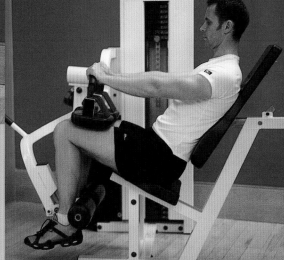

2 ▶ Hold your stomach tight and bend your legs, bringing your heels toward your butt. Hold for half a second, then slowly return to the start position. Exhale as you lift the weights and inhale as you lower them.

level			
repetitions	15 rm	15 rm	15 rm

squats

This exercise uses many of the muscles in the lower body. It works the thighs and buttocks as well as the lower leg muscles, abdominals, and lower back as they are used for balance. As you progress, use hand weights to increase the intensity of the exercise.

1 ▼ Stand with your feet hip-width apart. Keep your back straight and place your hands on your hips.

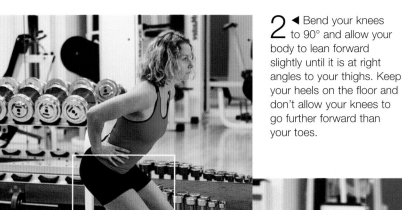

2 ◄ Bend your knees to 90° and allow your body to lean forward slightly until it is at right angles to your thighs. Keep your heels on the floor and don't allow your knees to go further forward than your toes.

3 ► Keep your back flat and use your lower leg muscles, abdominals, and lower back to balance. Squeeze your buttock muscles, then slowly return to the start position. Take care not to straighten the legs entirely at the top of the movement since this will lessen the effectiveness of the exercise. Breathe in as you lower your body down and breathe out as you push upward.

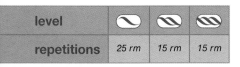

level			
repetitions	25 rm	15 rm	15 rm

lunges

A demanding exercise, the lunge works the muscles in the legs and hips and can give you wonderfully toned inner thighs and buttocks. Take two to three seconds on the way down and two to three seconds on the way up. Use hand weights to make the lunge more challenging.

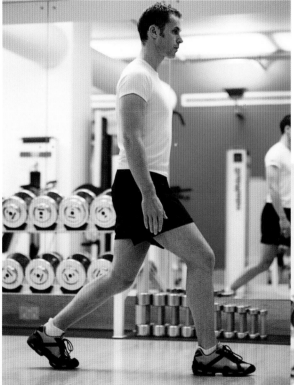

1 ◄ Place one foot forward about one stride length apart from the back leg, keeping your hips facing straight ahead and your arms loose by your sides. Keep your body upright and your abdominals firm.

2 ▼ Bend your knees to bring your front knee directly over your front foot. Concentrate on the movement being downward rather than forward; put your weight onto the heel of your front foot to work the buttock muscle most effectively. Raise yourself to the start position; repeat.

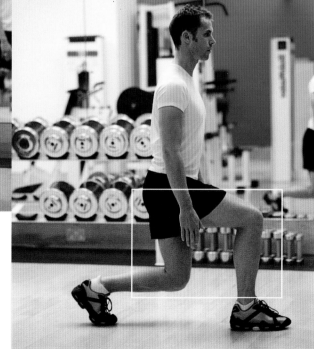

level	⬭	⬭	⬭
repetitions	25 rm each leg	25 rm each leg	20 rm each leg

push-ups

Push-ups use the weight of the body to work the triceps, pectorals, and deltoids (arm, chest, and shoulder muscles). Start with the half push-up and progress to the full push-up once you have built up strength.

1 ▶ Place your hands directly under your shoulders with your fingers pointing forward. Keep your torso and legs straight.

2 ▼ Bend your arms to about 90° and lower your body, keeping your head in line with your spine. Keep your stomach and thigh muscles tight, which will help to keep your legs straight. Be careful not to point your butt in the air. Push yourself back up to the start position. Remember to breathe in on the way down and out as you push up.

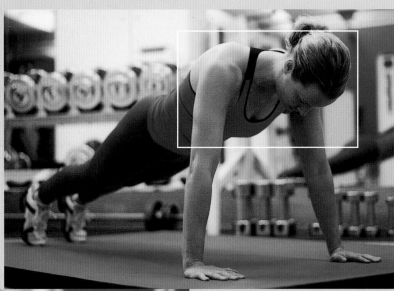

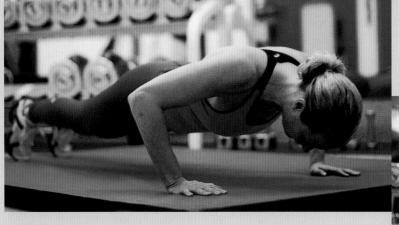

level	⬭	⬭	⬭
repetitions	15	20	30

▶ Or try the half push-up Keep arms in the same position as for the full push-up, but keep knees on the mat. Lower the body, then return to the start position.

lat pull-downs

This exercise works the large muscles of the back – the latissimus dorsi, or lats, and the rhomboids. Level three should do the more advanced pull-ups (*see below*).

1 ▶ Hold the handles of the machine so that your thumbs point behind you. Keep your back straight and your abdominals tight at all times.

2 ▼ Pull down and, as you do so, breathe out. Breathe in as you return to the start position. The whole exercise should take about 4 seconds.

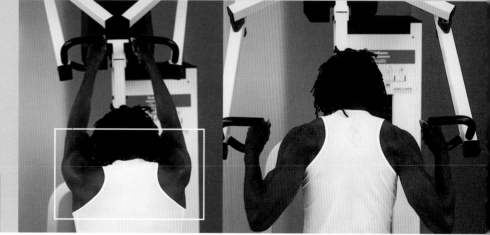

level			
repetitions	15 rm	15 rm	–

pull-ups

An excellent upper-body exercise, pull-ups are the definitive test of strength because you have to lift your own body weight. They work the biceps and back muscles and always look impressive.

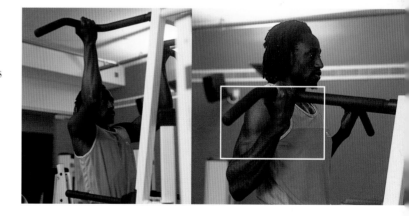

1 ▲ Hold the handles of the machine firmly. Take 2–3 seconds to pull yourself up until your shoulders are level with your hands. Breathe out with the effort and in as you return to the start position.

2 ▲ Take 2–3 seconds to lower yourself to the start position, but don't straighten your arms entirely. Keep your abdominals tight. Use the strength in your arms to stabilize you, or bend your knees beneath you.

level			
repetitions	–	–	10

bicep curls

level	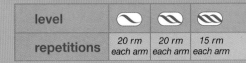		
repetitions	20 rm each arm	20 rm each arm	15 rm each arm

A great isolation exercise, the bicep curl gives fantastic definition to the upper arm.

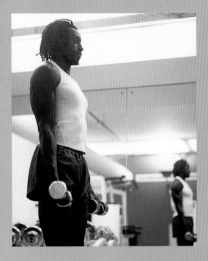

1 ◄ Stand with feet hip-width apart, knees slightly bent, and arms by your sides. Start with your elbows slightly bent and hold the weights so that your palms face forward.

2 ► Bend your elbow and lift the weight toward your shoulder. Keep your elbows tucked in close to your body. At the top of the movement, flex your bicep to maximize the effectiveness of the exercise. As you lower one arm, raise the other, and continue alternating arms, but do not allow your body to sway with the movement.

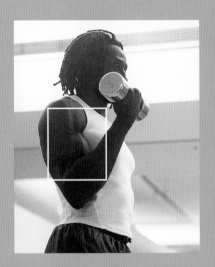

hammer curls

level	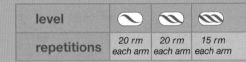		
repetitions	20 rm each arm	20 rm each arm	15 rm each arm

The hammer curl sculpts and tones the outer sections of the biceps and can actually make your arms appear longer.

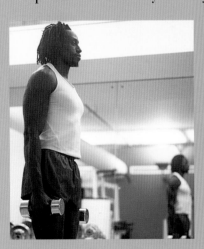

1 ◄ Stand with feet hip-width apart, legs slightly bent, and arms by your sides. Start with your arms slightly bent. Hold the weights so that your palms face inward.

2 ► Lift the weight toward your shoulder, keeping your elbows tucked in close to your body. Flex the bicep at the top of the movement, then return to the start position and repeat, alternating arms. Do not allow your body to sway with the movement.

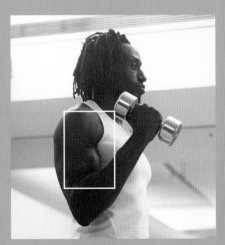

tricep extensions

The triceps are the muscles at the backs of the upper arms. Keep your abdominal muscles tight during the tricep extension as this will help you to stay in the correct position and maximize the effectiveness of the exercise.

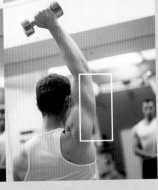

1 ▶ Rest your right hand and knee on a bench, keeping your left foot on the floor. With a dumbbell in your left hand, raise your elbow so that it is bent at 90° and your upper arm is parallel to the floor.

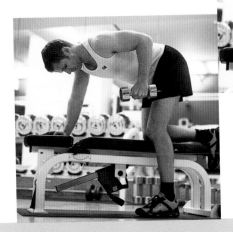

level			
repetitions	20 rm each arm	20 rm each arm	15 rm each arm

2 ▲ Hold the elbow position and straighten your arm while flexing the tricep. Slowly return to the start position. Take 4–5 seconds to complete the entire movement.

tricep overheads

This exercise is an alternative to tricep extensions (*see above*). If you find it difficult to keep your body steady while performing this exercise, try sitting upright on the end of a bench.

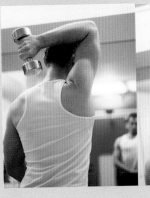
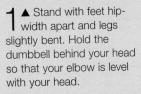

1 ▲ Stand with feet hip-width apart and legs slightly bent. Hold the dumbbell behind your head so that your elbow is level with your head.

2 ▲ Extend your arm, keeping your elbow close to your head and taking care not to let your elbow "drift" out of position. Keep your abdominal muscles tight to prevent straining the back. Slowly return to the start position.

level			
repetitions	20 rm each arm	20 rm each arm	15 rm each arm

85

chest press

level			
repetitions	20 rm	20 rm	15 rm

Using free weights for this exercise requires more muscle control than when using the chest-press machine.

1 ▼ Lie on your back on a bench with your knees bent and feet on the bench. Holding a weight in each hand, bend your arms so that your elbows are at 90° and your palms face the wall across from you.

2 ▼ Extend your arms upward so that they are nearly straight. Return to the start position, using a pace of about 4 seconds per repetition.

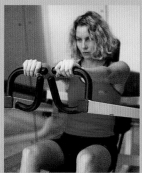

▲ Or try the gym alternative
Ensure that your lower back is supported. Push forward until your arms are almost straight, then bring your arms back until your elbows are level with your shoulders.

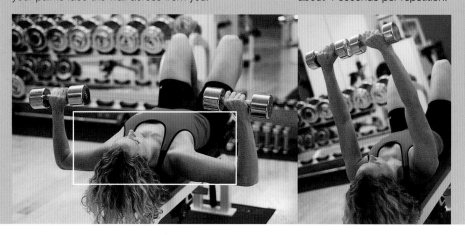

single arm row

Using the same body position as for the tricep extension (*see page 85*), here you lift a weight toward your body, working the biceps, backs of the shoulders, and upper back. Focus on using your bicep to lift the weight.

1 ▼ Rest your left hand and knee on a bench, keeping your right foot on the floor. Hold a dumbbell in your right hand; let your arm hang down toward the floor.

2 ▼ Your back should be parallel to the bench. Pull the dumbbell toward your chest, keeping your body stable, your back straight, and your shoulders relaxed. Return to the start position; keep the movement slow and controlled.

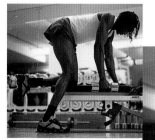

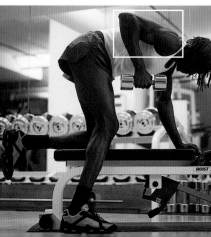

level			
repetitions	18 rm each arm	18 rm each arm	15 rm each arm

pec flys

This is the definitive exercise for the pectorals, or chest muscles. As always, good technique is crucial.

level	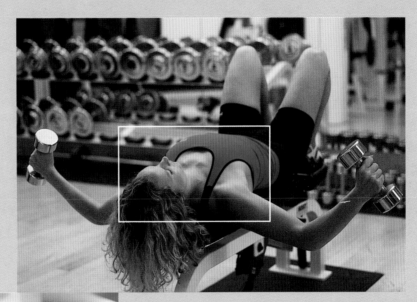		
repetitions	*15 rm*	*15 rm*	*10 rm*

1 ▶ Lie on your back on a bench with your knees bent and feet on the bench. Holding a weight in each hand with your palms facing the wall across from you, extend your arms out away from your sides until your hands are level with your shoulders.

2 ▼ While breathing out, use your chest muscles to slowly raise the weights up until your arms are nearly fully extended above your chest. Flex your pectorals, then, breathing in, slowly return to the start position.

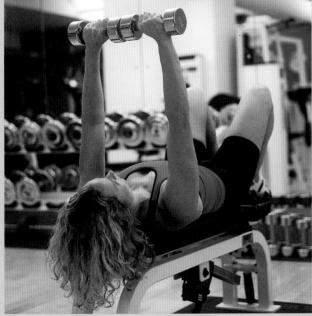

▼ **Or try the gym alternative** Focus on using your pectorals rather than your arms to push the bars together. Keep your head and neck relaxed and your back upright and straight.

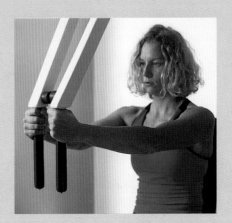

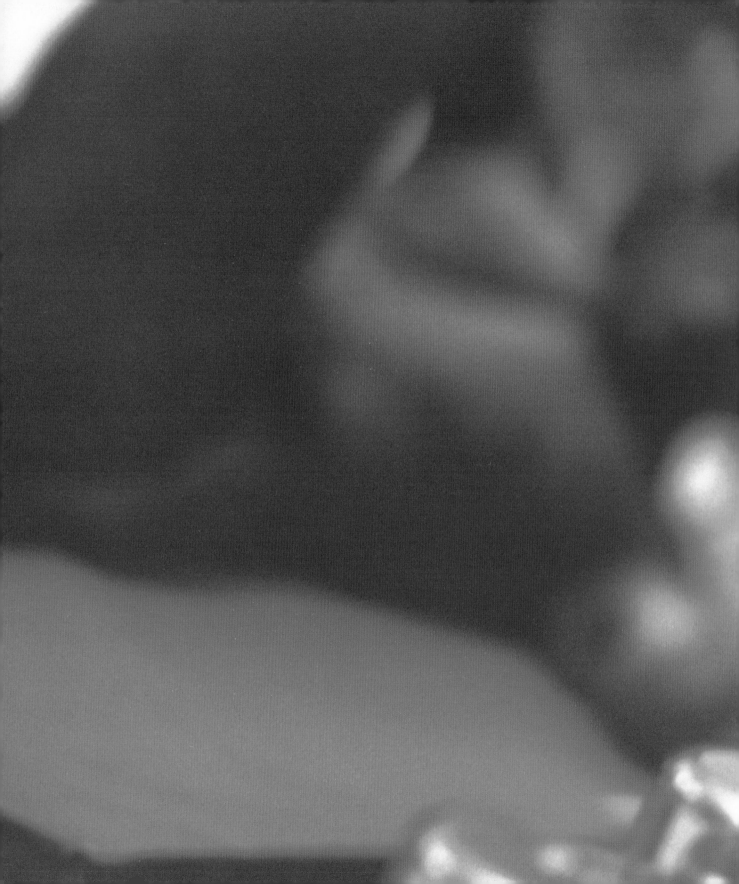

phase two

push

By now you should be feeling stronger and

yourself

more confident. In Phase Two, you use your

increased energy levels to further develop

your cardiovascular health, tone the muscles,

and increase your metabolic rate. Spend 21

days on this phase.

nutritional goals

By now you should be on course with the goals set in Phase One. Keep up the good work. In Phase Two we add more goals: here we tackle lunch. As so many of us fit it into a busy day and eat it away from home, it is often the most difficult meal to control.

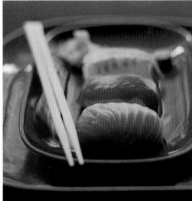

sushi – healthy and increasingly easy to find

lunch goals
• Eat lunch every day, and eat it half-way through the day at a regular lunchtime, not midway into the afternoon
• Limit lunches containing wheat to two per week

phase 2 goals
• Limit tea and coffee intake to two cups in total per day

tea and coffee
Both tea and coffee dehydrate the body. Since one of the main aims of the detox is to keep the body well hydrated so it can function at optimum efficiency, drinking large amounts of tea and coffee will not help achieve the desired effects. Substitute herbal teas or, ideally, water.

lunch
Take time out at lunchtime and relax while you eat. Chew your food thoroughly as this breaks it down earlier in the digestive process and enables the body to extract more nutrients from it. Try not to drink too much with your meal since this flushes the food through the body more quickly and prevents the body from digesting it as thoroughly. Drink most of your water mid-morning and mid-afternoon.

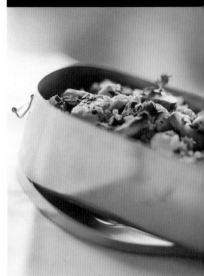

if you can find time, make your own lunch

Lunch should be the most filling of your daily meals. At this time of day, the body is in full swing. A good lunch raises the metabolic rate and provides the body with the energy it needs to sustain it for the remainder of the day. Try to eat complex carbohydrates such as rice, root vegetables, couscous, and pasta as they are slow releasers of energy and ensure that you won't experience energy highs and lows during the afternoon.

what makes a healthy lunch?

If you can find time, try to make your own lunch (*see panel*). When buying any pre-prepared food, check the saturated fat content. Fat content should be no higher than 15 percent, of which saturates should make up no more than 5 percent of the total calories.

All too often we reach for convenience food at lunchtime, and the obvious choice is the sandwich. The sandwich can be a healthy option, but look out for the following.

• The bread. Go for organic wholemeal bread, although rye bread is a tasty wheat-free option. Wholemeal bread is the least processed and the least acid-forming (*see pages 70–1*), and is less likely to give you a sugar rush, which means you won't need a snack in the afternoon.

• The filling. Avoid cheese and hidden calories in the form of mayonnaise, butter, and margarine. Try a salad filling with fish or chicken.

healthy lunches

Rice salads Easy to prepare yourself: boil the rice with a little stock; add fresh herbs and chopped vegetables such as peppers, broccoli, and mushrooms.

Sushi A healthy option, increasingly popular and even sold in some supermarkets.

Raw vegetables with dips Try carrots, celery, cucumber, broccoli, and cauliflower, for example; experiment with dips such as hummus and tzatziki; beware of reduced fat varieties – they may still be high in fat.

Fresh salad Experiment with leaves and vegetables of your choice; try adding pumpkin or sesame seeds; avoid cheese or mayonnaise dressings.

Couscous salad Make your own: add any combination of sliced grilled chicken breast, chick peas, and vegetables such as steamed or grilled zucchini, eggplant, onion or peppers, and fresh mint.

Wholemeal pasta salads Try cooked pasta with vegetables such as broccoli, spinach and snow peas, and fresh herbs.

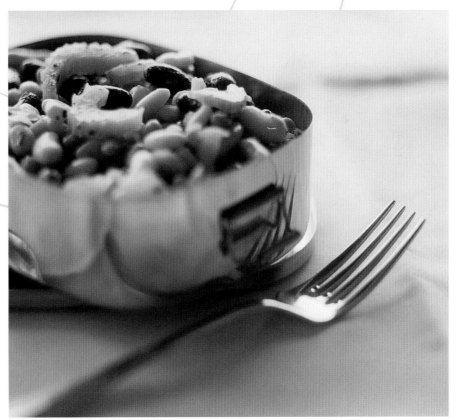

bean salad – a great wheat-free option

aerobic training

In Phase Two, you build on your improved level of aerobic endurance and continue to develop your cardiovascular system. Here you work your heart and lungs and build stamina using interval training, which works the body at different levels – a more difficult level followed by a period of recovery.

The frequency of exercise in Phase Two is four times per week for all groups. The exercise is performed at two levels of intensity, with the higher level being the most challenging. Work at the higher level for the time specified, then slow down so that your heart rate drops to the lower level. Allow yourself to recover at this level for the time specified, then take the intensity back up to the higher level.

    This two-stage workout is done four times to give you a total workout time of 20 minutes training in your optimum training zone. Before you begin exercising, remember to start with a five-minute low-intensity warm-up, then do some warm-up stretches (*see pages 44–5*).

phase 2 aerobic training chart

level			
frequency	4 per week	4 per week	4 per week
intensity	75% MHR for 3 mins 70% MHR for 2 mins	85% MHR for 3 mins 70% MHR for 2 mins	90% MHR for 3 mins 75% MHR for 2 mins
perform	4 times	4 times	4 times
total time	20 mins	20 mins	20 mins

resistance training

In Phase Two, you train using peripheral heart action (PHA), which works the muscles as well as conditioning the heart. Follow two of your weekly aerobic training sessions with the resistance training program below. Once you are familiar with the exercises (*see pages 94–9*), photocopy this page and refer to it in the gym.

It is important that you perform the exercises in the order in which they are listed below. The exercises alternate between lower and upper body so the heart is constantly having to work to keep blood flowing up and down the body. This strengthens the heart as it is forced to work at a challenging pace.

Work through the exercises from start to finish, then repeat the sequence until you have completed the number of circuits specified for your fitness level at the bottom of the chart.

phase 2 resistance training chart

level			
leg press	25 rm	25 rm	25 rm
push-ups	max	max	max
power lunges	30	40	50
lateral raises	15 rm	15 rm	12 rm
bicep curls	20 rm	40 rm	60 rm
step-ups	20	25	30
leg curls	15 rm	15 rm	12 rm
chest press	15 rm	12 rm	12 rm
basic crunch	10	15	20
reverse curl	10	15	20
full crunch	10	15	20
rest for	2 minutes	2 minutes	2 minutes
perform	3 circuits	4 circuits	5 circuits

resistance exercises

The principle behind peripheral heart action training is to work the upper and lower body in quick succession. This tones the muscles, but also strengthens the heart.

leg press

This exercise tones the glutes (butt) and the quads (the muscles at the fronts of the thighs). Keep checking technique; even small errors can put strain on the back and knees.

level	◔	◑	◕
repetitions	25 rm	25 rm	25 rm

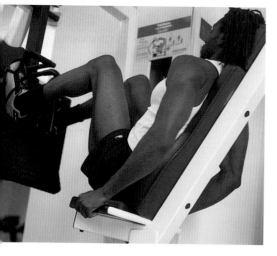

1 ◄ Start with your knees bent at 90°, feet about shoulder-width apart. Hold the handles at the side of the machine and make sure that your lower back is supported at all times.

2 ► Push against the foot plate, with about 70% pressure on the heels and 30% on the toes. Push, squeezing your buttock muscles, until your knees are almost, but not entirely, straight. Return to the start position, using your thigh muscles for control. Breathe out as you push and breathe in on your return. Take 2 seconds to push and 2–3 seconds to return.

► **Or try this** Position a stability ball between your lower back and the wall. Keep your back straight and slowly lower yourself, as if sitting down on an imaginary chair, until your knees are bent at 90°. Slowly roll back up the wall.

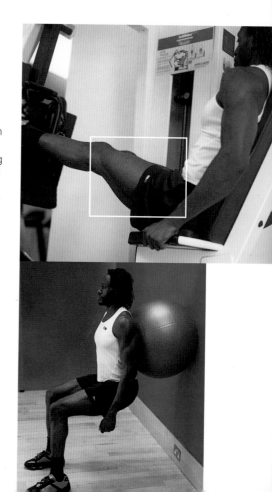

push-ups

▶ When performing the full push-up, keep your abdominals tight, your body straight, and your head in line with your spine. If you can't hold the correct position, return to the easier half push-up until you have built up adequate strength. **For push-ups, see page 82.**

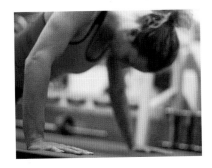

level	⬭	⬭	⬭
repetitions	*max*	*max*	*max*

power lunges

A more dynamic version of the lunge (*see page 81*), the power lunge works the quads and hamstrings (the leg muscles) and the glutes (the butt). These are quicker than the lunge, but the movement should still be steady and controlled.

level	⬭	⬭	⬭
repetitions	30	40	50

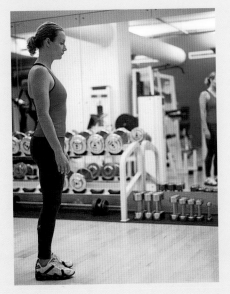

1 ◀ Stand with feet hip-width apart, arms loose by your sides.

2 ▶ Step forward about one stride length apart from the back foot, making sure that your knee does not bend further forward than your toes. As you do so, lower your body down, then spring back to the starting position, pushing through with the heel of your front foot. Keep your arms loose by your sides, and do not allow your body to waver.

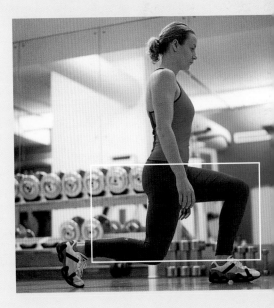

lateral raises

Keep your arms parallel to the floor in the finish position, to ensure that you work all three sections of the deltoid, or shoulder muscle, evenly.

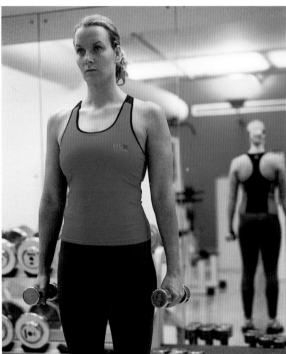

1 ◄ Stand with feet hip-width apart, knees slightly bent. Start with your arms by your sides, holding dumbbells so that your palms face inward. Keep your abdominals tight.

level			
repetitions	15 rm	15 rm	12

2 ► Slowly lift your arms away from your sides, keeping your elbows slightly bent, until your hands are at shoulder level. Keep your palms facing downward; don't allow your hands to twist. Keep your torso still – if it moves, you are using your body to lift the weights and not your deltoids. Take about 2 seconds to lift the weights and 2 seconds to lower them, breathing out as you lift and in as you lower.

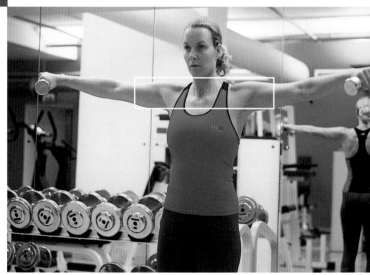

bicep curls

▶ If you find that your body sways with the momentum of lifting the dumbbells, you may need to go down in weight. Correct technique is more important than the weight of your dumbbells. **For bicep curls, see page 84.**

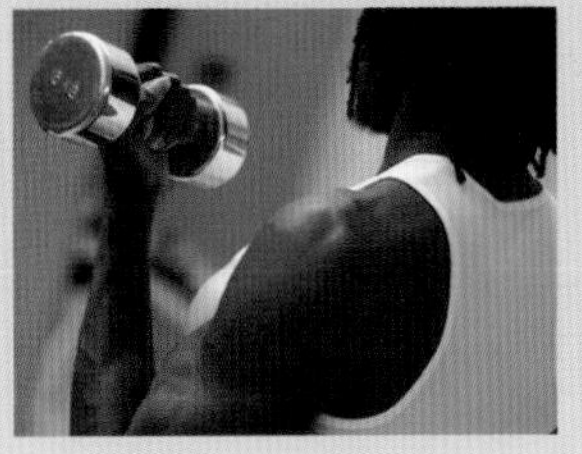

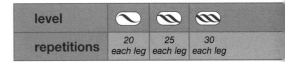

level			
repetitions	*20 rm each arm*	*40 rm each arm*	*60 rm each arm*

step-ups

Go briskly through this exercise: step-ups work your lower body muscles, but they should also raise your heart rate.

level			
repetitions	*20 each leg*	*25 each leg*	*30 each leg*

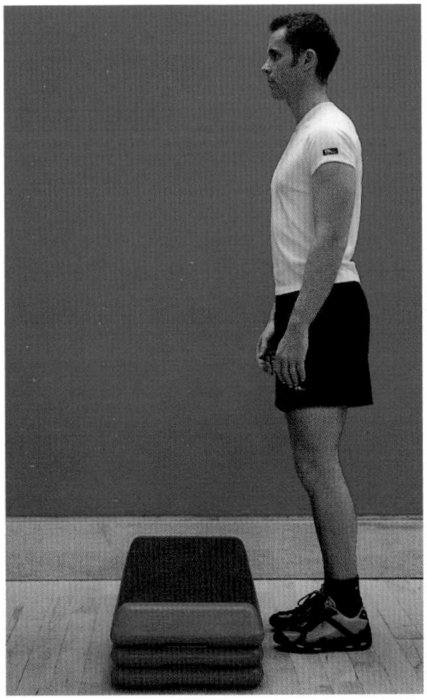

1 ▲ Adjust the step so that your knee does not bend to less than 90° when you step on to it. Stand facing the step, arms by your sides.

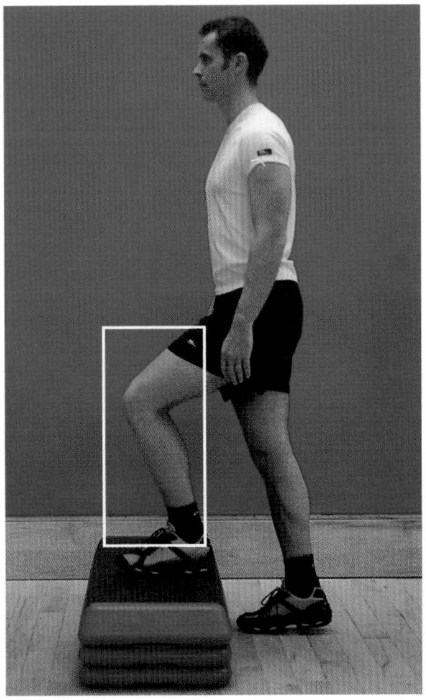

2 ▲ Step up with one foot, placing your whole foot flat on the step. Keep your back straight and your head and neck relaxed but in line with your torso.

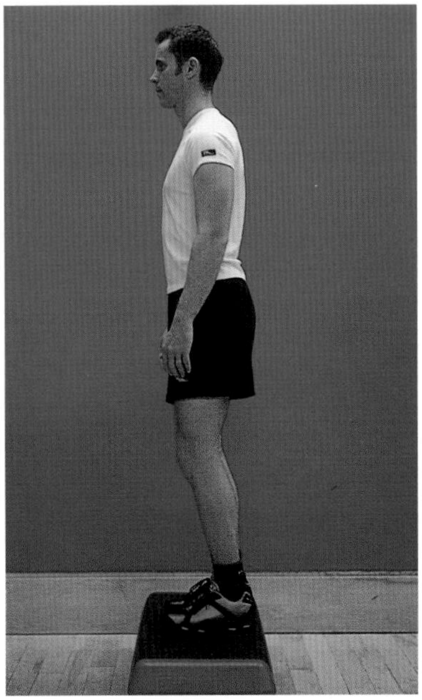

3 ▲ Step up with your other foot so that both feet are flat on the step. Step down one foot at a time: land on your toes first, then roll the foot down until the heel touches the ground.

leg curls

▶ Get the most out of the leg curl by holding the finish position for about half a second before returning to the start position. **For leg curls, see page 79.**

level			
repetitions	*15 rm*	*15 rm*	*12 rm*

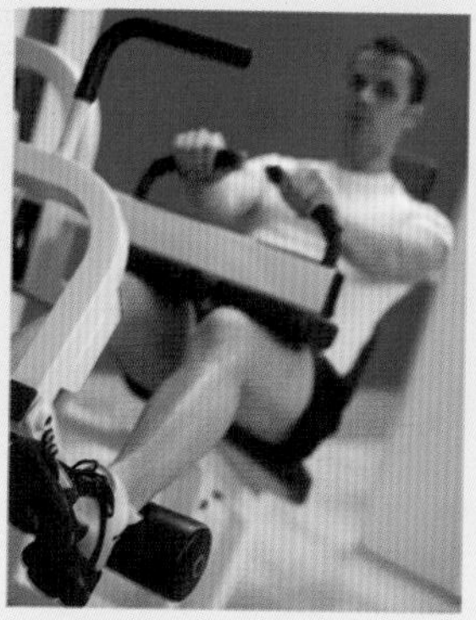

chest press

▶ Keep the movement for the chest press slow and controlled, taking about 4 seconds per repetition. **For chest presses, see page 86.**

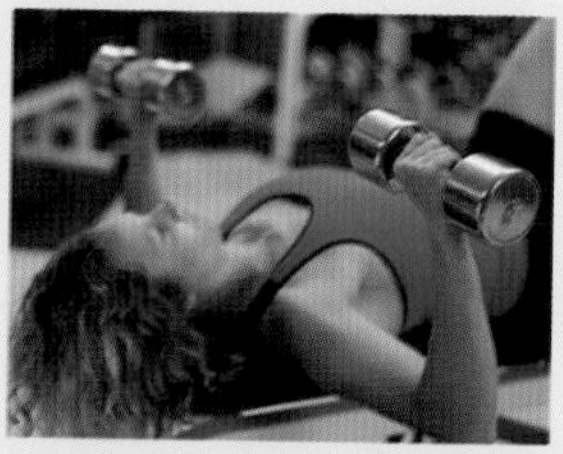

level			
repetitions	*15 rm*	*12 rm*	*12 rm*

basic crunches

Of all the abdominal exercises, the basic crunch is one of the most effective. The key is to keep the movement slow and to focus on good technique.

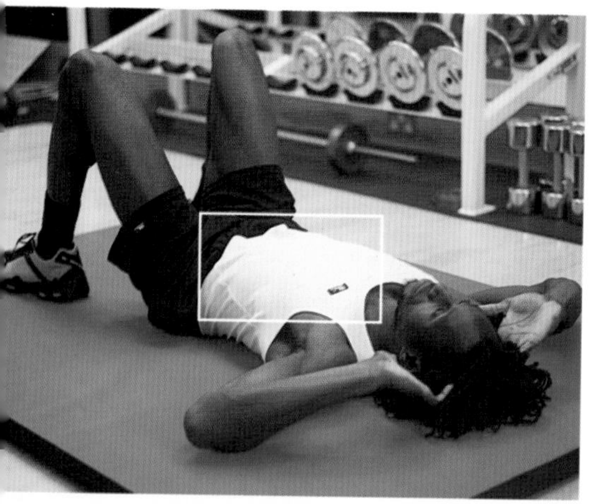

level			
repetitions	*10*	*15*	*20*

1 ◀ Lie on your back with your knees bent, feet flat on the floor and hands by your ears.

2 ▶ Curl your shoulders forward, keeping your lower back on the floor. Tense the abdominals, breathing out as you lift and in as you lower. Keep a space the size of an apple under your chin, to ensure that your head stays in line with your spine. Each repetition should take about 4–5 seconds.

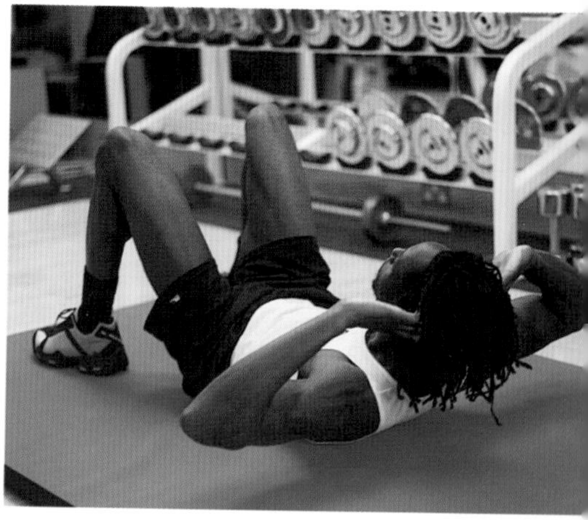

reverse curls

Many people find that the reverse curl puts less strain on the neck area than the basic crunch (*see opposite*).

level	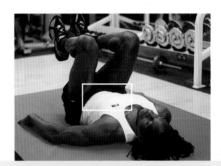		
repetitions	10	15	20

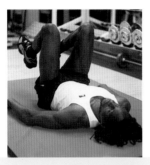

1 ◀ Lie on your back with your arms by your sides, legs in the air, and knees bent. Keep your shoulders and head on the floor at all times. Ensure that your knees never go further back than directly over the hips.

2 ▶ Tighten your lower abdominals and curl your legs and pelvis toward your ribcage. Keep your upper legs at 90° to your torso – pulling your knees too close to your head can strain your lower back.

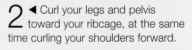

full crunches

The most advanced abdominal exercise, this combines the movements of the basic crunch (*see opposite*) and the reverse curl (*see above*) and works the whole stomach area.

level	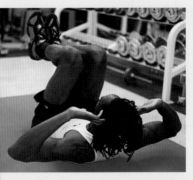		
repetitions	10	15	20

1 ▼ Lie on your back with your legs in the air, knees bent, and hands either side of your head by your ears.

2 ◀ Curl your legs and pelvis toward your ribcage, at the same time curling your shoulders forward.

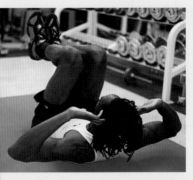

▶ **Or try this** Lie with a stability ball positioned under your lower back, your hands crossed over your chest and your feet flat on the floor. Curl your body up slightly, until your abdominals are tight.

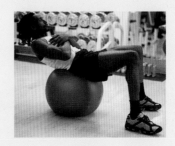

retest yourself

You should have been following the program for 42 days, or six weeks, now. This marks a natural point to pause, consider your achievements, and assess your progress.

taking stock

By now, if you are on course with the program and achieving your goals, you should have begun to see changes to your body shape and to feel a noticeable improvement in your general well-being. Do you feel as though you have lost weight, changed shape, or become stronger? If you have not begun to see real physical results yet, this does not mean that you are not making progress. At this stage, you should be starting to notice two fundamental changes:

• You should feel much more energetic.
• You should feel much more self-confident.

the benefits so far

If you were hoping to have lost a lot of weight, you will be disappointed; but that is because you set yourself an unrealistic goal. You certainly should not expect to see excessive weight loss – no health program should advocate massive weight loss in this length of time. A safe rate at which to lose weight – and to lose it permanently – is about one to two pounds (half to one kilogram) a week.

    The simple fact that you are feeling better should empower you and will bring you closer to your goals. The increase in energy levels is an indication that your body has begun to detoxify. It is a sign that your body is beginning to use your energy reserves more efficiently. The interval training that was introduced in Phase Two will have helped to increase your aerobic capacity, that is the level at which your body can take in oxygen and use it efficiently. You will have raised your basal metabolic rate and learned how to overload your body, or push it beyond

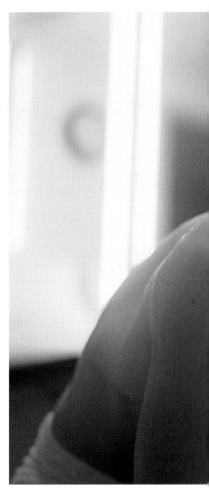

pause to take stock

its normal limits, and it will be burning calories more quickly as a result. You will also have increased your overall muscle utilization so your muscles are working more efficiently and burning more energy – the ultimate effect of this is that you burn more fat. You will probably have lost some weight; you will certainly have lost some body fat, and as a result, you should be noticing changes to your body shape.

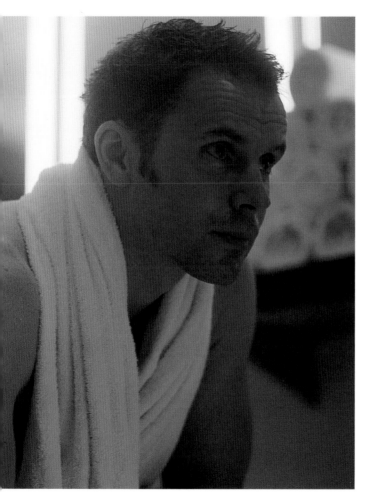

the importance of retesting

Your body has begun to adjust to the program. Turn back to pages 30–35 and do the physical, nutritional, and personality questionnaires again, then compare your new scores with your original ones.

It is very important that you monitor your progress. You must be aware of the changes that your body is undergoing. Retesting enables you to respond to changes – positive or negative. The more you see results, the more they will fuel your motivation. If you have retested and found a marked improvement, well done; but try not to become complacent. Aim to continue with the same level of dedication. Don't be tempted to change level mid-program. By all means experiment with the exercises for the level above, but continue to work at your own level because the program is going to become more challenging.

If you have seen no improvement, have you been following the program closely enough? The stricter you are with yourself and the stronger your resolve to stay with the program, the closer I can get to guaranteeing that it will work. If you have been faithful to it and have still not seen results, talk to your doctor and explain what you have been doing. It is unusual for a person to feel no benefits at all from the program.

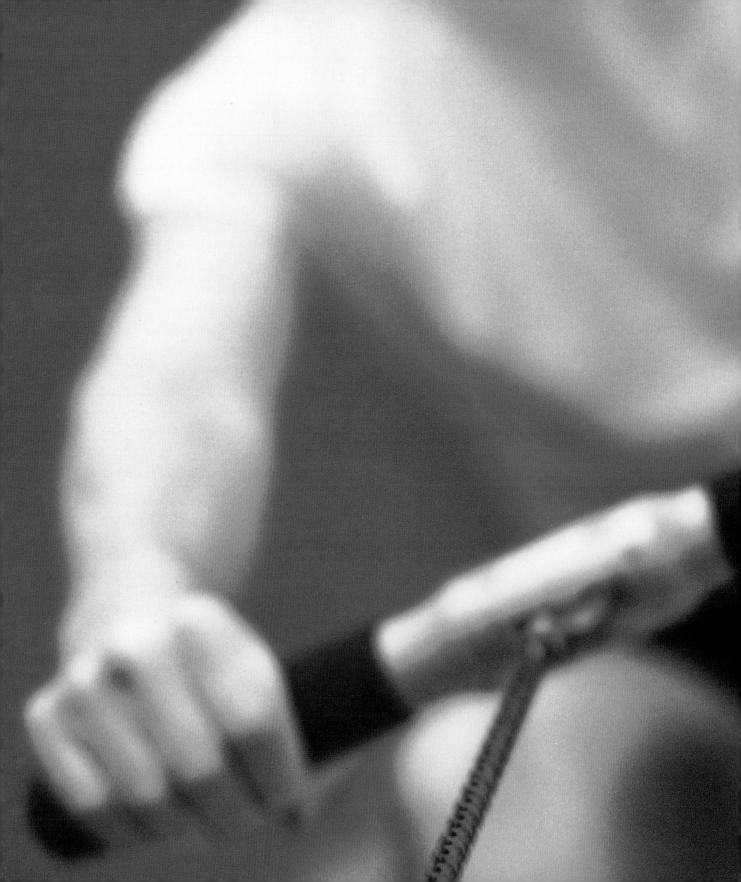

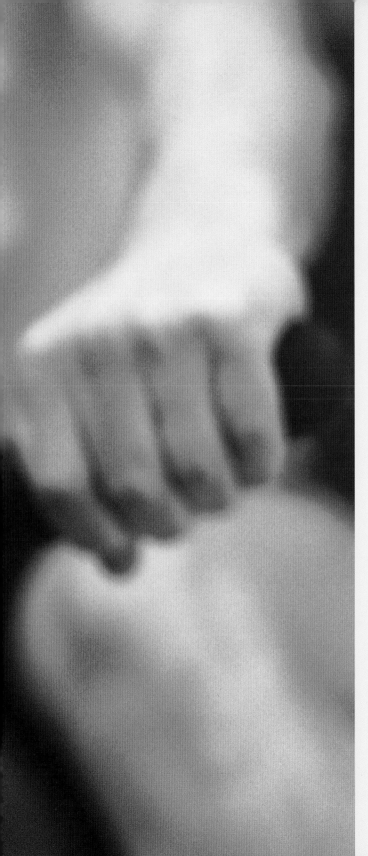

phase three

extending

In Phase Three, you build upon the improved level

your

of fitness that you will have attained by now.

base

Extended periods of aerobic training will increase

your endurance, and the circuit resistance training

will improve your stamina. Take 14 days to

complete this phase.

nutritional goals

By now you should have breakfast under control and be experimenting with a variety of different lunches. You should also be drinking plenty of water and eating lots of fresh fruit and vegetables. All this will be helping to cleanse your system and make you stronger and more energetic.

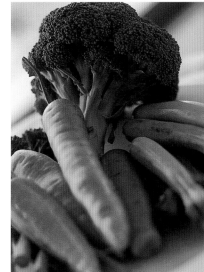

eat more fresh vegetables

dinner goals
• Try to eat as early in the evening as possible, preferably at least two hours before you go to bed
• Reduce the size of your evening meal and aim to make it less starchy

phase 3 goals
• Make sure that only one of your meals each day contains wheat products such as bread, pasta, and couscous
• Increase your intake of dark green vegetables

less wheat
Wheat is not the most digestion-friendly food, and by now you should be adjusting to eating less of it, replacing it with more fresh fruit and vegetables. Begin to phase wheat out of your evening meals now and experiment with replacements such as wild rice, beans, millet, lentils, and barley. These have a cleansing effect on the body because of their high fiber content and are an excellent source of protein, which the body needs to maintain and repair itself. You can also buy wheat-free pasta and bread.

dinner
The earlier in the evening you eat, the better. This allows the body time to digest food properly, while you are awake and active. If you eat and go to bed soon after, it does not have enough time to digest what you have eaten before resting.

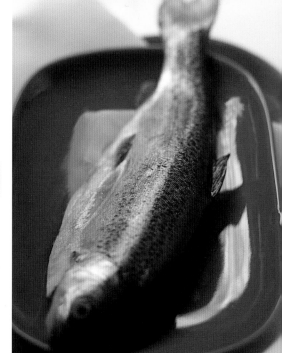

the fat in fish is good for you

Food sits in the body overnight, then passes out without being properly digested, or it can hang around too long in the body as undigested waste.

When you can't eat early in the evening, make sure that the later you eat, the more alkaline the meal (*see pages 70–1*), since alkaline foods are easier to digest. If you know that you are going to eat less than two hours before going to bed, have a meal that does not contain meat, wheat, or dairy products since these acid-forming foods are more difficult to digest. This way you are working with your body to give it what it needs when it needs it.

eat your greens

Children are told to eat their greens, and the same applies to adults. Vegetables such as broccoli, spinach, kale, zucchini, and asparagus all have antioxidant properties, as do red peppers and carrots. Antioxidants are our first line of defense against aging, heart disease, cancer, and the harmful effects of stress. They neutralize free radicals, unstable substances that occur in the body as a by-product of oxidation, which can cause damage, especially to cell membranes.

size is important

The body needs more energy during the day, when you are active, and less energy during the night, when you are asleep. Alter the size of your meals accordingly: make breakfast and lunch your bigger, heartier meals and keep your evening meal simple and more alkaline-based (*see panel for suggestions*). Try to include protein, vegetables, and occasionally some carbohydrates. Enhance the flavor of food by experimenting with fresh herbs and spices rather than cooking with fat and oil. Remember that the fat in fish is good for you as it contains selenium, an antioxidant, which can help control cholesterol levels and may also help protect against cancer.

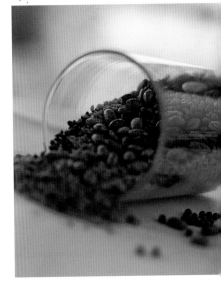
experiment with beans and lentils

healthy dinners

Grilled or steamed fish
Oily fish high in Omega-3 fatty acids are best: try trout, salmon, sea bass, tuna, and mackerel.

Seasonal vegetables Eat them raw, steamed, or roasted.

Vegetable risotto Try mushroom, zucchini, or asparagus, but do not include cream or cheese.

Stir-fries Vegetables such as snow peas, bean sprouts, carrots, onion, and peppers can be combined with shrimp or skinned chicken breast; use a small amount of oil and cook quickly to ensure the vegetables stay crunchy.

Beans and lentils Try bean soup or dahl.

Frozen yogurt and sorbet These are good low-fat dessert options.

Fruit Try fresh fruit salad, poached pears, or baked apples instead of desserts made with lots of sugar and cream.

aerobic training

This is where you really begin to challenge the body. With your improved levels of fitness and confidence, you should also feel that you have built your aerobic capacity up to a level where it can cope with the extra intensity required in this phase.

In Phase Three you return to building your aerobic endurance levels, but here you work for longer periods of time and at a greater intensity. This is far more challenging than Phase One endurance training. Levels one and two train aerobically three times a week, while level three does so four times a week.

Your total workout times will vary with each weekly session; some workouts will be more difficult than others. Keep checking your heart rate as you work. By now, you will find that you have to work harder than before to achieve the same heart rates. This is an indication that you have greatly improved your level of fitness.

phase 3 aerobic training chart

level			
frequency	3 per week	3 per week	4 per week
intensity	70-80% MHR	80-85% MHR	80-85% MHR
time	1 x 30 mins per week 2 x 40 mins per week	1 x 30 mins per week 2 x 45 mins per week	1 x 40 mins per week 2 x 45-50 mins per week 1 x 60 mins per week

resistance training

In Phase Three you use circuit training as a method of resistance training, performing a series of exercises in a specified time, rather than working with reps. The circuits appear on pages 108–11 and should be performed twice a week to work both the upper and lower body. Take a photocopy of this page to the gym for easy reference.

Circuit training tones the muscles while keeping the heart rate elevated so there is also a cardiovascular benefit. Take care not to let your technique suffer as you work more quickly than usual. Once you have completed one circuit, take your timed rest period, then continue to work through the circuits, resting in between, until you have completed the required number. Do both circuits once a week after two of your aerobic training sessions.

phase 3 resistance training charts
upper body circuit

level			
push-ups	30 secs	45 secs	60 secs
crunches	30 secs	45 secs	60 secs
shoulder press	30 secs	45 secs	60 secs
step-ups	30 secs	45 secs	60 secs
bicep curls	30 secs	45 secs	60 secs
shuttle runs	30 secs	45 secs	60 secs
ball pass	30 secs	45 secs	60 secs
lateral raise	30 secs	45 secs	60 secs
rest	60 secs	60 secs	90 secs
perform	5 circuits	5 circuits	5 circuits

lower body circuit

level			
squats	45 secs	60 secs	60 secs
shuttle runs	45 secs	60 secs	60 secs
full crunches	45 secs	60 secs	60 secs
step-ups	45 secs	60 secs	60 secs
side strides	45 secs	60 secs	60 secs
push-ups	45 secs	60 secs	60 secs
jog on the spot (high knees)	45 secs	60 secs	60 secs
rest	90 secs	90 secs	60 secs
perform	4 circuits	4 circuits	5 circuits

upper body circuit

This eight-exercise circuit focuses on working the muscles in the upper body. It includes aerobic exercise to help vary the pace and work the heart and lungs. All levels complete the circuit five times.

push-ups

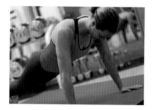

1 ◄ Keep your hands positioned directly under your shoulders, your back straight, and your head in line with your spine. **For push-ups, see page 82.**

level	◎	◎	◎
seconds	30	45	60

crunches

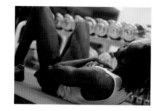

2 ◄ Count 3 seconds as you lift and 3 seconds as you lower. Crossing the arms over the chest makes the exercise slightly easier. **For crunches, see pages 98–9.**

level	◎	◎	◎
seconds	30	45	60

shoulder press

This exercise works the deltoids, or shoulder muscles. It can also be performed using dumbbells.

level	◎	◎	◎
seconds	30 rm	45 rm	60 rm

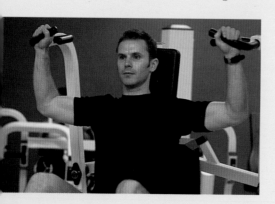

3 ◄ Hold the handles so that your elbows are bent at 90°. Keep your abdominals tight and your lower back supported at all times.

▶ Lift the weights by pushing the handles above your head. Exhale as you push, taking care not to lock your arms straight. Breathe in as you return to the start position.

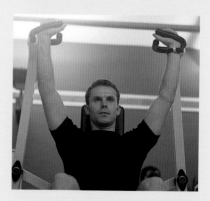

step-ups

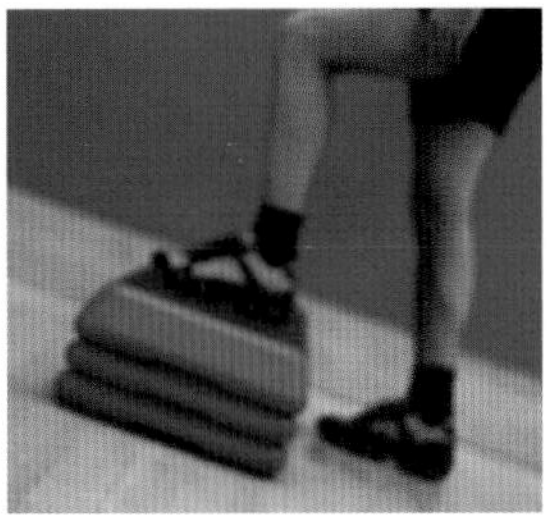

4 ▶ Take care not to let your knee bend to less than 90° when you step up as this can strain it. **For step-ups, see page 97.**

level			
seconds	30	45	60

bicep curls

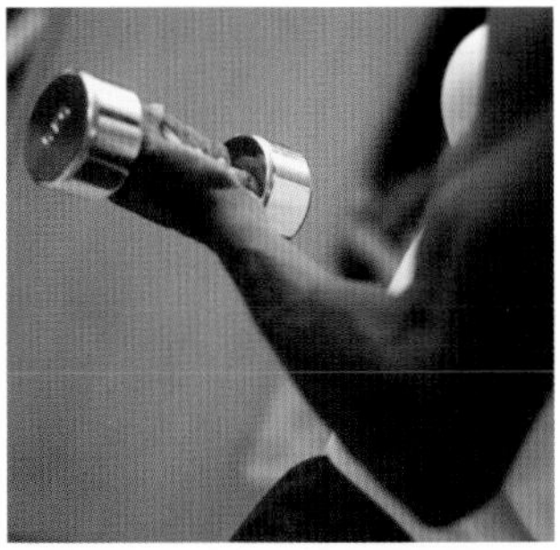

5 ◀ Focus on using your bicep to lift the weight. Keep the movement slow and controlled to maximize the effectiveness of the exercise. **For bicep curls, see page 84.**

level			
seconds	30	45	60

shuttle runs

6 ▶ Place 2 markers 30ft (10m) apart. Run between the markers, planting one foot at right angles to each marker to provide a strong base to pivot off as you turn around.

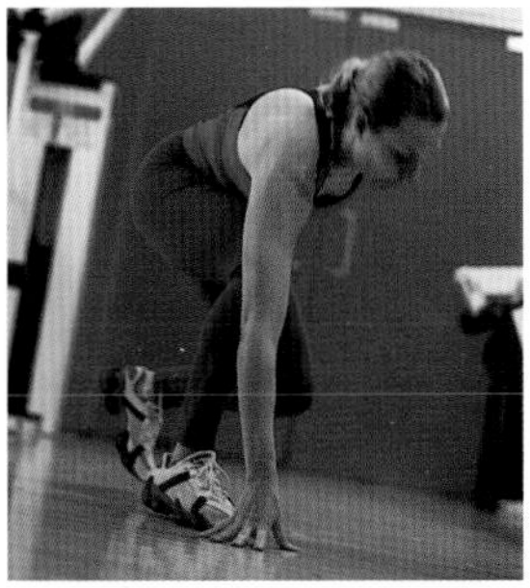

level			
seconds	30	45	60

ball pass

level			
seconds	30	45	60

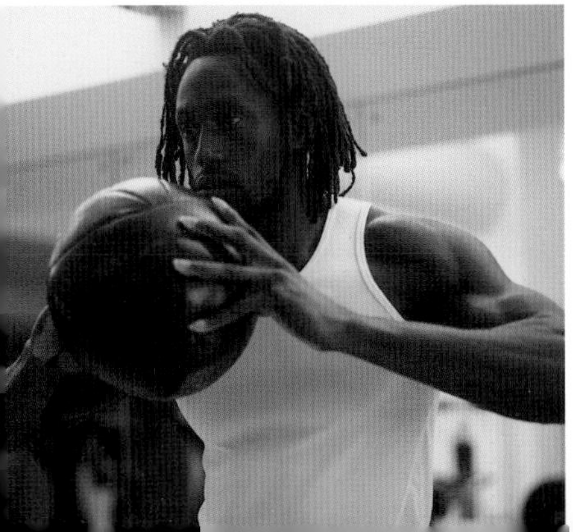

7 ◀ Use a medicine ball for this exercise. Stand slightly further than arm's length away from a wall, legs shoulder-width apart. Hold the ball at chest level with elbows out by sides. Throw the ball against the wall, pushing straight out from your chest. Pull the ball back into your chest as you catch it. Repeat.

lateral raise

8 ▶ Keep your back straight and your abdominals tight. Take care not to allow your back to arch or your hands to twist. **For lateral raises, see page 96.**

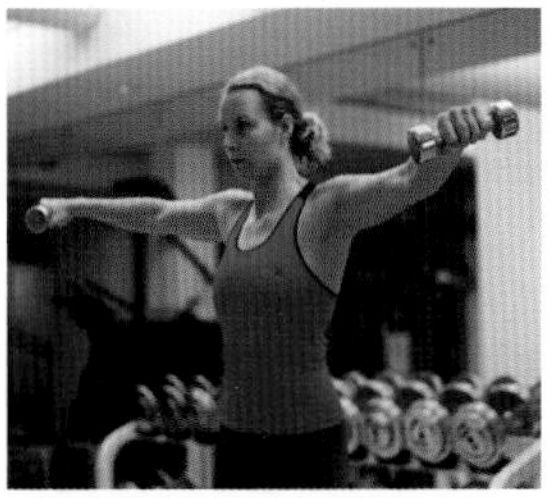

level			
seconds	30	45	60

lower body circuit

This seven-exercise circuit works the large muscles of the legs. Work quickly, but take care not to sacrifice technique. Levels one and two should do four circuits, level three should do five.

squats

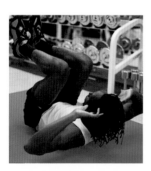

1 ◄ Take care not to let your back arch or your heels lift off the floor when performing squats. **For squats, see page 80.**

level	⬭	⬭	⬭
seconds	45	60	60

shuttle runs

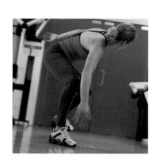

2 ► Make shuttle runs more difficult by increasing your range of movement and lifting your knees to waist height when running. **For shuttle runs, see page 109.**

level	⬭	⬭	⬭
seconds	45	60	60

full crunches

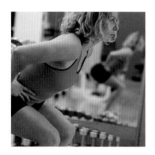

3 ◄ Keep the movement slow and controlled, and concentrate on using your abdominals to complete the full crunch. Keep your head in line with your spine. **For full crunches, see page 99.**

level	⬭	⬭	⬭
seconds	45	60	60

step-ups

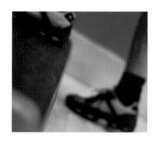

4 ► Keep checking your posture: your back should be upright and your head and neck should be relaxed as you step up and down. **For step-ups, see page 97.**

level	⬭	⬭	⬭
seconds	45	60	60

side strides

This exercise increases the heart rate and works the muscles of the inner and outer thigh. Move quickly, and complete as many as possible in the time specified for your level.

level	◔	◑	◕
seconds	45	60	60

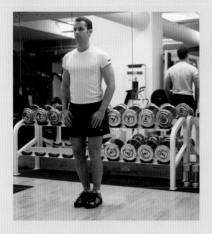
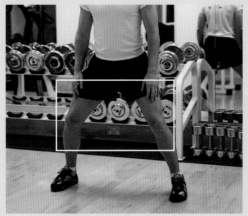
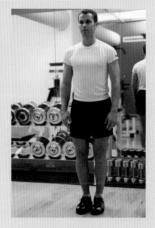

5 ▲ Stand with feet together, abdominals tight and arms by your sides.

▲ Step sideways. Ensure that you keep your back straight.

▲ Complete the movement by bringing your feet together. Step sideways the other way and repeat.

push-ups

6 ▶ Keep your stomach and thigh muscles tight during full push-ups as this will help to keep your legs straight. Breathe in as you lower yourself down and out as you push up. **For push-ups, see page 82.**

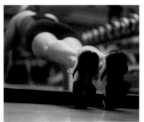

level	◔	◑	◕
seconds	45	60	60

jog on the spot

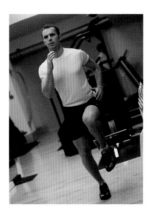

7 ◀ Lift your knees to waist height and keep your abdominals tight as you jog in place. Land on your toes; your heel should touch down only briefly during the movement.

level	◔	◑	◕
seconds	45	60	60

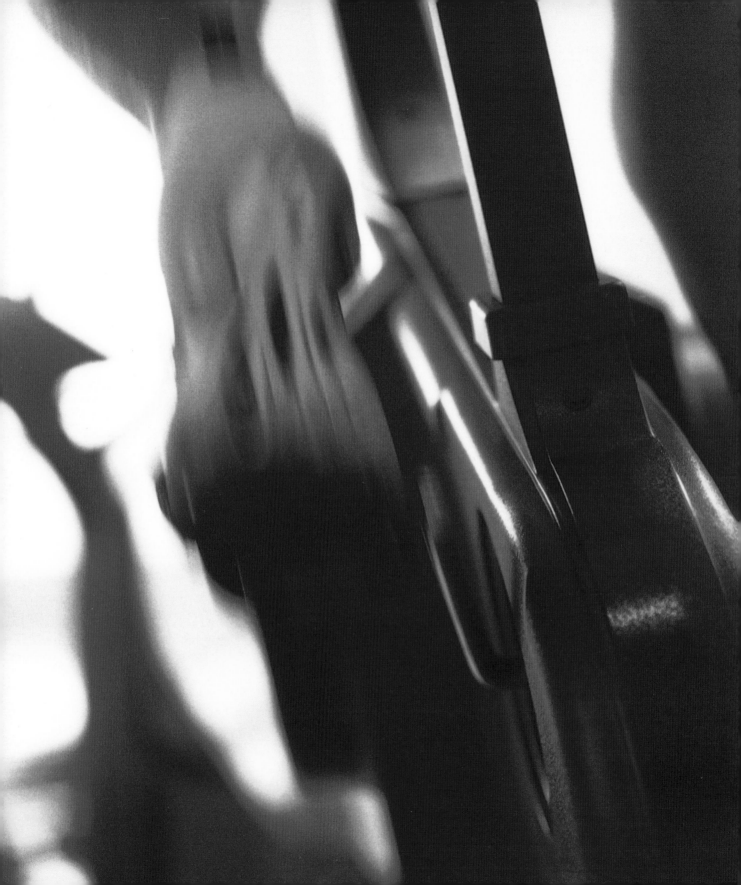

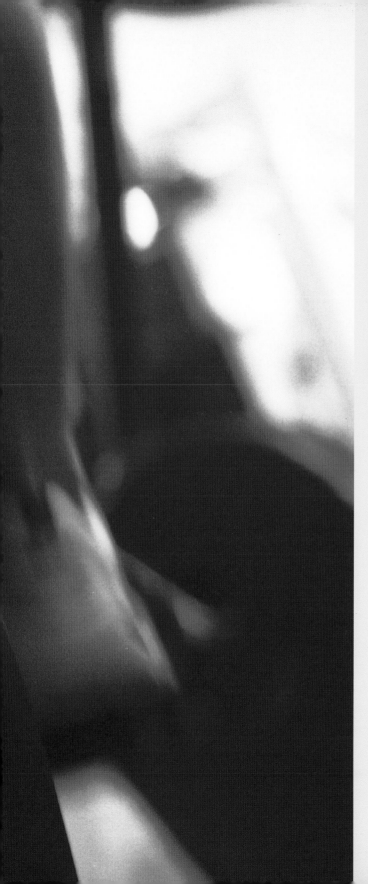

phase four

becoming

Your higher level of fitness and the positive

an

changes in your body shape should be keeping

advanced

you motivated and on course. In Phase Four,

exerciser

you continue to challenge the body and

introduce variety into your training regime.

Spend 21 days on this phase.

nutritional goals

You've worked hard to reach this point, and hopefully it hasn't been too difficult. The aim has been to make big changes to your diet, but gradually, without shocking the body. You have cleansed your system and you should really feel the positive effects as your body begins to function more efficiently. You should be achieving all the goals in Phase Four by now.

snack goals

- Eat small quantities of low-fat, low-sugar foods
- Snack when hungry, not when bored

phase 4 goals

- Drink 3–4 pints (1.5–2 liters) of water a day
- Eat wheat products at only one meal a day
- Reduce dairy product intake where possible
- Eat four pieces of fruit a day
- Eat at least three portions of vegetables every day
- Build variety into all meals
- Eat as much raw food as possible, or steam, grill, or stir-fry, to keep the goodness in
- Chew your food thoroughly
- Take time to sit down and enjoy food
- Eat a lunch packed with energy foods such as vegetables, rice, couscous, and wholemeal pasta every day
- Eat dinner early, and when you eat later, eat more alkaline foods
- Eat mainly alkaline-forming foods

snacks

Recent research carried out in the US found that the average person eats approximately 23 lb (10.5 kg) of snacks a year, and as a nation, the US spends a total of $13.4 billion on snack foods. Now, 50 percent of Americans are considered obese. People are getting fatter because they eat more and exercise less.

Snacking is important because it helps to regulate the body's blood sugar levels. Through the program's nutritional goals, you

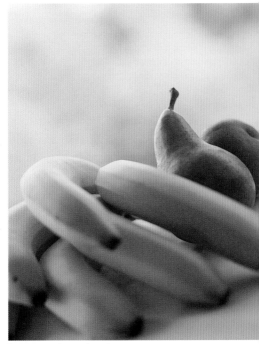

bananas and pears boost energy

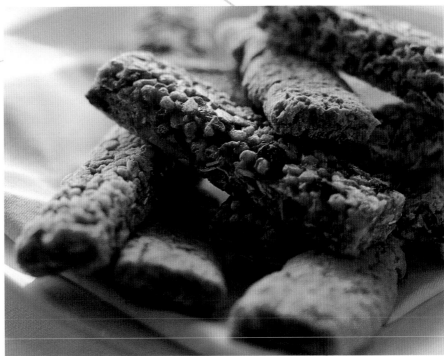

low-fat snack bars may not be as healthy as they look

healthy snacks

Nuts A great snack and a good source of protein; high in calories, so eat only in small amounts; choose pecans, almonds, hazelnuts, and walnuts; go for natural, unsalted varieties.

Seeds Pumpkin and sunflower seeds are high in protein, zinc, iron, vitamin E, and phosphorus, they boost energy and promote healthy skin and bones; zinc can help boost fertility levels in men; relatively low in calories.

Fresh fruit Keep fruit close at hand so when you are tempted to snack, you are more likely to reach for a healthy option; pears and bananas are good sources of potassium and boost energy.

Dried fruit Higher in natural sugar than fresh fruit so should be eaten in smaller quantities, but still a good source of nutrients. Try figs, raisins, prunes, and apricots: good sources of vitamin C, antioxidant, and high in soluble fiber; check they are free from mineral oil and artificial preservatives.

have introduced more slow-release energy foods into your diet – that is foods that deliver a constant supply of energy over a long period of time. This means that you shouldn't experience energy lows that make you crave sugary foods for the quick-fix energy highs they provide. If your body becomes accustomed to a diet high in processed sugar, you will get used to snacking and then craving another snack an hour later to revive your flagging energy levels. Eating alkaline foods prevents this roller-coaster effect of blood sugar highs and lows.

the truth about low-fat snack bars

We carried out our own research and bought 15 different low-fat snack bars from retailers. Over 60 percent of them had more than 35 percent sugar content. These bars were low in fat but very high in sugar and had little nutritional value. They simply lock you into a cycle of craving. Read labels: by law, they should list the ingredients in order of quantity, starting with the greatest.

aerobic training

In Phase Four, your improved level of fitness enables you to alter the emphasis of your training and concentrate on making more cosmetic changes to your body shape.

By now, you should be noticing a dramatic improvement in your level of fitness; you should be finding that you have to work much harder to raise your heart rate to the desired level. Once you do reach it, the aim is to keep your heart rate elevated for the entire period specified for each workout.

    The time for which you train has been reduced in this phase compared to the time in Phase Three. This is to enable you to put more of your energy into the resistance side of the workout.

phase 4 aerobic training chart

level			
frequency	3 per week	4 per week	5 per week
intensity	70% MHR	75% MHR	80% MHR
time	25 mins	23-35 mins	45-60 mins

resistance training

The aim of Phase Four is to sculpt and tone the body and define the muscles. The exercises appear on pages 118–21. Photocopy this page to use as reference at the gym.

phase 4 resistance training chart

level	⬭	⬭	⬭
chest press	12 rm	10 rm	8 rm
pec flys	12 rm	10 rm	8 rm
tricep overheads	12 rm	10 rm	10 rm
slow push-ups	-	max (2 secs up, 2 secs down)	max (5 secs up, 1 sec down)
perform	3 sets	3 sets	3 sets
lat pull-downs	12 rm	10 rm	8 rm
bicep curls	12 rm	10 rm	10 rm
upright row	12 rm	10 rm	8 rm
single arm row	-	12 rm	10 rm
perform	3 sets	3 sets	4 sets
leg extension	12 rm	10 rm	10 rm
leg curl	12 rm	12 rm	10 rm
leg press	12 rm	12 rm	12 rm
lunges	20 rm	15 rm	15 rm
perform	3 sets	3 sets	3 sets
lateral raise	12 rm	10 rm	10 rm
shoulder press	12 rm	12 rm	10 rm
perform	3 sets	4 sets	4 sets

Here, you tone the muscles by increasing the intensity of your workout, using medium weights and high repetitions.

The number of sets specified at the end of each sequence of exercises refers to the whole sequence; do each series of exercises, then repeat the sequence until you have completed the required number of sets. Complete the specified number of sets for each sequence before you move on to the next sequence.

Do this workout after any two of your weekly aerobic training sessions. Cool down at the end of your aerobic training session, then follow the resistance training program in the chart. Remember to cool down at the end of your workout (*see pages 46–7*).

resistance exercises

In Phase Four we decrease the number of repetitions and increase the resistance to define the muscles and give a toned athletic appearance to the body. For each exercise sequence, do the number of sets specified for your fitness level (*see page 117*).

chest press

1 ▶ As you return to the start position, bring your elbows back so that they are level with the shoulder joint and no further. **For chest press, see page 86.**

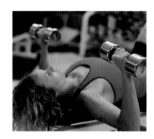

level	⬯	⬯	⬯
repetitions	12 rm	10 rm	8 rm

pec flys

2 ▶ Keep your elbows slightly bent as you raise your arms and focus on generating movement from your shoulders. **For pec flys, see page 87.**

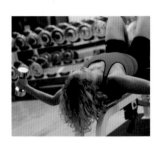

level	⬯	⬯	⬯
repetitions	12 rm	10 rm	8 rm

tricep overheads

3 ▶ Hold your abdominals tight to prevent straining the back, and keep the movement slow and controlled. **For tricep overheads, see page 85.**

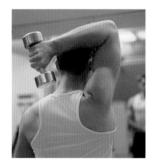

level	⬯	⬯	⬯
repetitions	12 rm each arm	10 rm each arm	10 rm each arm

slow push-ups

4 ▶ This is a more intense version of the standard push-up. Level two should count 2 seconds up and 2 seconds down. Level 3 should count 5 seconds up and 1 second down. **For push-ups, see page 82.**

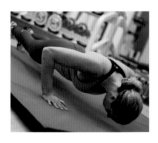

level	⬯	⬯	⬯
repetitions	-	max	max

lat pull-downs

1 ▶ A common mistake is to allow the back to arch as you pull down. This can put serious strain on the back, but it will also make the exercise less effective. **For lat pull-downs, see page 83.**

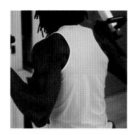

level	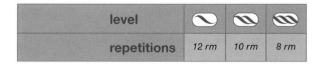		
repetitions	12 rm	10 rm	8 rm

bicep curls

2 ▶ Keep your elbows close to your body. Lower the weight, but don't straighten your arm completely at the end of the movement. **For bicep curls, see page 84.**

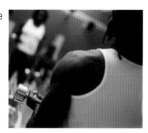

level			
repetitions	12 rm each arm	10 rm each arm	10 rm each arm

upright row

This is a good exercise for the deltoids, or shoulder muscles, and the biceps, the muscles at the front of the upper arms. It can be performed using dumbbells or a bar.

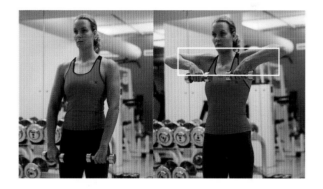

level			
repetitions	12 rm	10 rm	8 rm

3 ▲ Stand with feet hip-width apart, legs slightly bent, and back straight. Hold the weights in front of you so that your palms face your thighs.

▲ Pull the weights up to chest height, leading with the elbows. Slowly lower the weights and return to the start position.

single arm row

level			
repetitions	-	12 rm each arm	10 rm each arm

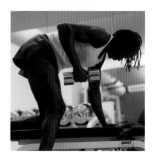

4 ◀ Keep your back straight and concentrate on lifting the weight straight up toward your chest with a slow and controlled movement. Pull through with the elbow so that it comes back, behind the body. **For single arm row, see page 86.**

leg extension

leg curl

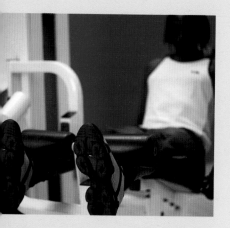

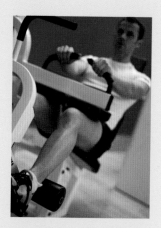

1 ◄ Keep your movement slow and controlled to get the most from this exercise. Count 3 seconds as you lift, then hold the finish position for half a second and count 3 seconds to return to the start position. **For leg extensions, see page 78.**

2 ► The most common mistake with the leg curl is to allow the back to bend in the finish position. This can put enormous strain on the lower back, but it also takes the emphasis away from the hamstrings. **For leg curls, see page 79.**

level			
repetitions	12 rm	10 rm	10 rm

level			
repetitions	12 rm	12 rm	10 rm

leg press

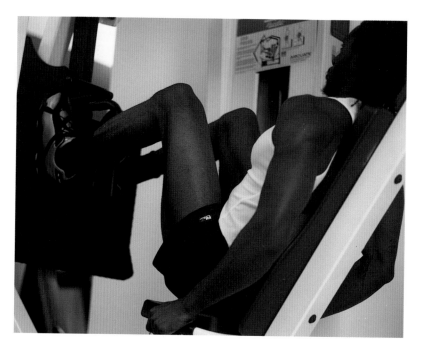

3 ► Breathe out with the effort as you push and in as you return to the start position. Use your thigh muscles to keep the movement slow and controlled. Ensure that your lower back is well supported. **For leg presses, see page 94.**

level			
repetitions	12 rm	12 rm	12 rm

lunges

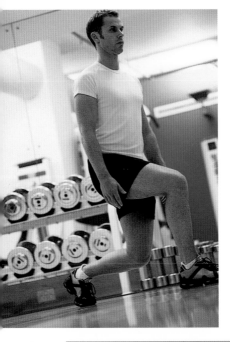

4 ◀ You can make this exercise more difficult by holding hand weights. Take care not to allow the knee to bend too far over the front of the foot as you lunge. **For lunges, see page 81.**

level			
repetitions	20 rm each leg	15 rm each leg	15 rm each leg

lateral raise

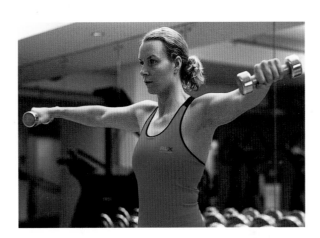

1 ▲ Lift your arms away from your sides until they reach shoulder level. Keep your elbows very slighty bent at all times. **For lateral raises, see page 96.**

level			
repetitions	12 rm	10 rm	10 rm

shoulder presses

2 ▶ Start with your elbows at shoulder height, arms bent at 90° so that hands are at head height. Push straight up, taking care not to lock your arms straight.

level			
repetitions	12 rm	12 rm	10 rm

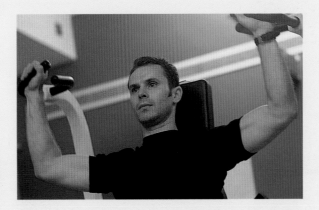

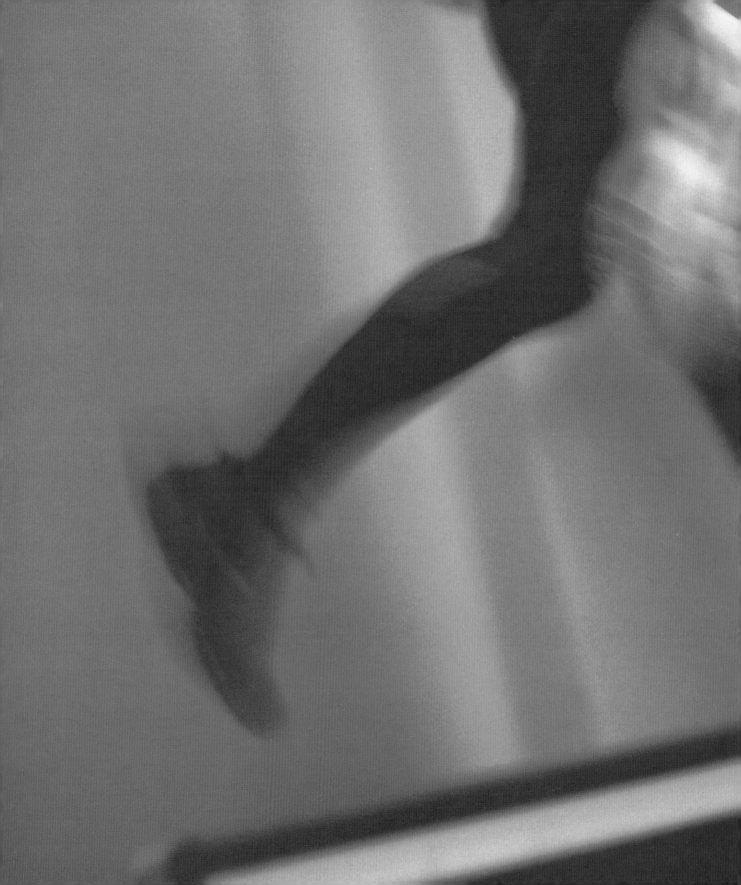

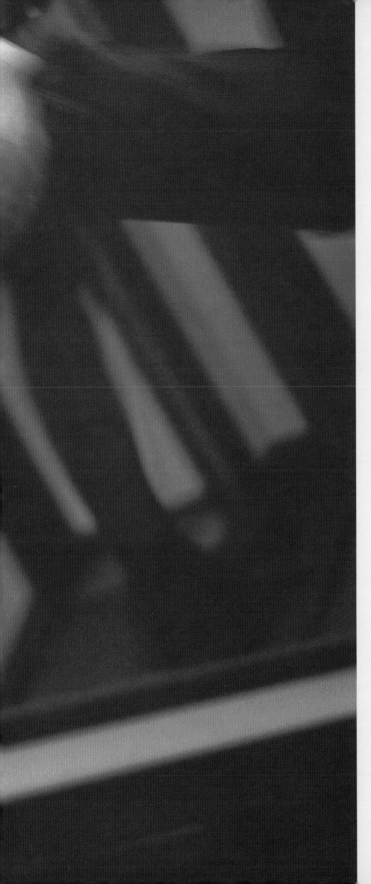

phase five

reaching

This is the fine-tuning phase of the program – and

your

also its most intensive part. The training

goals

techniques in this phase help to sculpt and shape

the body and achieve a healthy athletic look. Take

14 days to complete this phase, using the final day

to assess your progress and define new goals.

nutritional goals

By now you have made many beneficial changes to your diet in the course of the program. Continue with this new way of eating and try not to slip back into bad habits.

essential superfoods

Try to include as many as possible of these highly nutritious superfoods in your diet:

• **Apples** Rich in vitamin C, high in soluble fiber; can help relieve constipation and diarrhea and also benefit the circulation; help to keep blood sugar levels stable; an excellent alkaline-forming food; green apples are usually higher in vitamin C than red ones.

• **Bananas** Rich in potassium and magnesium; the starch and soluble fiber in bananas make them a good energy food; effective in the treatment of constipation and diarrhea; eating a ripe banana 30 minutes after exercise will help the body to recover.

• **Blueberries** Very rich in vitamin C, an antioxidant, which can help to strengthen the immune system.

• **Melon** Rich in vitamin C and potassium; one of the most alkaline foods, it balances acid in the digestive system.

• **Pineapple** High in fiber, rich in the enzyme bromelain, which breaks down protein, making it a valuable digestive aid; maintains a healthy heart and can help healing and tissue repair after injury.

• **Strawberries** Excellent source of vitamin C; high in soluble fiber; their antioxidant properties may help to protect against arthritis, anemia, and cancer.

• **Asparagus** Rich in vitamin C, beta-carotene, and selenium; helps with water retention.

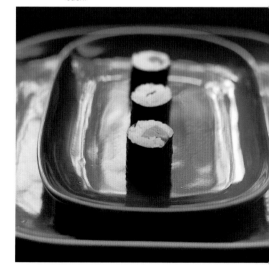

sushi

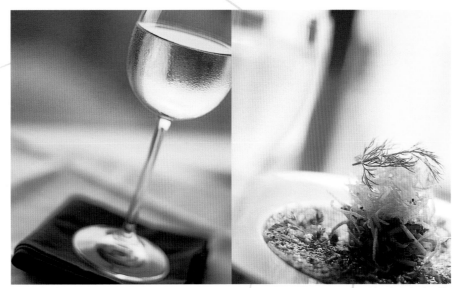

wine – fine in moderation   *restaurant food can be healthy*

healthy ideas for eating out

Poultry and game Order grilled or roast chicken, turkey, pheasant, or guinea fowl, but not duck, which is more fatty.

Fish and shellfish Order it steamed, grilled, baked, or flash fried; sushi, sashimi, and tuna carpaccio are all good, nutritious options

Light sauces Choose vegetable coulis, salsas, light tomato or yogurt-based sauces over rich, oily, or buttery ones.

Vegetables Ask for them to be steamed, stir fried, grilled, or lightly boiled so they are still crunchy.

Fried foods Order food that is flash fried not deep fried.

No butter Ask for food to be cooked without butter; it is often added to vegetables before they are served, and added to fish and meat before grilling.

Bread Stop yourself from absentmindedly filling up on bread at the start of a meal.

- **Carrots** Rich source of beta-carotene, an antioxidant; can help to lower blood cholesterol levels and maintain healthy skin, eyes, and heart.
- **Broccoli** Good source of beta-carotene, calcium, folic acid, and zinc; helps fight fatigue and stress; may help protect against cancer.
- **Oily Fish** Rich in protein, calcium, vitamin D, and Omega-3 fatty acids; can help control blood cholesterol levels; maintains healthy skin and hair.
- **Wild Rice** A nutrient-rich grass; high in protein, vitamin B, and zinc.

alcohol

The body identifies alcohol as a toxin, but that doesn't mean that it can't be enjoyed in moderation. Stick to one type of alcohol and try to drink it alongside equal quantities of water. I think that red wine is better than white wine, partly because it is generally matured for longer and so is less acidic, but also because it is more likely to have antioxidant properties because of the tannins in red grapes. Try to avoid beer as it is highly caloric and the calories are empty ones that will be stored as fat.

aerobic training

Follow the programs for endurance training, interval training, and circuit training, below.

phase 5 endurance training chart

level	◠	◠	◠
frequency	1 per week	1 per week	1 per week
intensity	85% MHR	85% MHR	85% MHR
time	30 mins	40 mins	45 mins

phase 5 interval training chart

level	◠	◠	◠
frequency	2 per week	2 per week	2 per week
intensity	75% for 1 min 90% for 1 min	75% for 1 min 90% for 1 min	75% for 1 min 90% for 1 min
perform	12 times	14 times	15 times
total time	24 mins	28 mins	30 mins

phase 5 circuit training

Do the lower body circuit training routine in Phase Three (*see pages 110–11*) once.

resistance training

phase 5 pyramid training chart

level	◠			◠					◠				
leg press	Set 1 15 rm	Set 2 12 rm	Set 3 15 rm	Set 1 15 rm	Set 2 12 rm	Set 3 10 rm	Set 4 12 rm	Set 5 15 rm	Set 1 15 rm	Set 2 12 rm	Set 3 10 rm	Set 4 12 rm	Set 5 15 rm
chest press	Set 1 15 rm	Set 2 12 rm	Set 3 15 rm	Set 1 15 rm	Set 2 12 rm	Set 3 10 rm	Set 4 12 rm	Set 5 15 rm	Set 1 15 rm	Set 2 12 rm	Set 3 10 rm	Set 4 12 rm	Set 5 15 rm
lat pull-down	Set 1 15 rm	Set 2 12 rm	Set 3 15 rm	Set 1 15 rm	Set 2 12 rm	Set 3 10 rm	Set 4 12 rm	Set 5 15 rm	Set 1 15 rm	Set 2 12 rm	Set 3 10 rm	Set 4 12 rm	Set 5 15 rm
leg curl	Set 1 15 rm	Set 2 12 rm	Set 3 15 rm	Set 1 15 rm	Set 2 12 rm	Set 3 10 rm	Set 4 12 rm	Set 5 15 rm	Set 1 15 rm	Set 2 12 rm	Set 3 10 rm	Set 4 12 rm	Set 5 15 rm

phase 5 compound training chart

Levels one and two, do a three-exercise sequence; level three, add a drop set as the fourth set, where weight is reduced to 75% of the first weight and the exercise performed until muscle fatigue. The figures in the chart refer to the exercises on pages 128–29.

level	◠	◠	◠
shoulders	1, 2, 3	1, 2, 3	1, 2, 3, 4
thighs	5, 6, 7	5, 6, 7	5, 6, 7, 8
triceps	9, 10, 11	9, 10, 11	9, 10, 11, 12
biceps	13, 14, 15	13, 14, 15	13, 14, 15, 16

pyramid training

This training method works with either three- or five-set workouts. The aim is to make the workout harder, by increasing the weight used, by the second or third set. The weights are then lowered in the last one or two sets.

leg press

1 ▶ Use your thigh muscles to control the movement. Breathe out with the effort as you push and in on your return. **For leg presses, see page 94.**

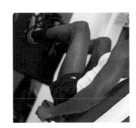

level	⬭	⬭	⬭
repetitions	*3 sets*	*5 sets*	*5 sets*

chest press

2 ▶ Take care not to bend your elbows beyond 90° when you return to the start position. **For chest presses, see page 86.**

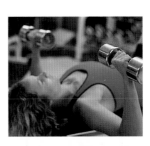

level	⬭	⬭	⬭
repetitions	*3 sets*	*5 sets*	*5 sets*

lat pull-down

3 ▶ Keep your back straight and take care not to lean forward as you pull down. **For lat pull-downs, see page 83.**

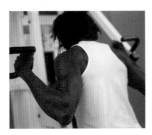

level	⬭	⬭	⬭
repetitions	*3 sets*	*5 sets*	*5 sets*

leg curl

4 ▶ Keep your abdominals tight and your lower back supported throughout this exercise. **For leg curls, see page 79.**

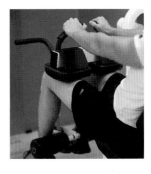

level	⬭	⬭	⬭
repetitions	*5 sets*	*5 sets*	*5 sets*

compound training

Levels one and two do three-exercise sequences. Level three add a drop set as the fourth set where they do an exercise until overload is reached, then drop to 75 percent of the initial weight and continue until overload is achieved a second time.

shoulders

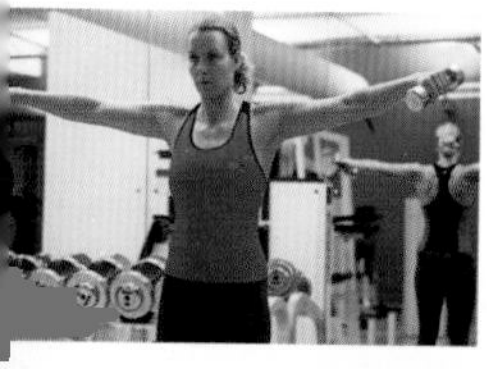

1 ◀ **Lateral raise** Take care not to twist the dumbbells as you raise your arms. **For lateral raises, see page 96.**

level			
repetitions	14–16 rm	12–14 rm	10–12 rm

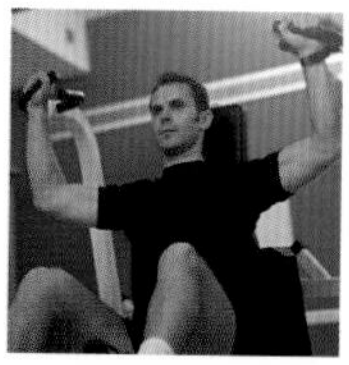

2 ◀ **Shoulder press** Breathe out with the effort and in as you lower the weight. **For shoulder presses, see page 108.**

level			
repetitions	14–16 rm	12–14 rm	10–12 rm

3 ▶ **Upright row** Keep the dumbbells close to your body as you pull up. **For upright row, see page 119.**

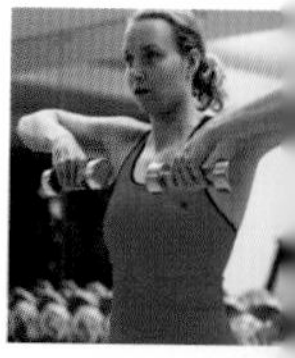

level			
repetitions	14–16 rm	12–14 rm	10–12 rm

4 ▼ **Lateral raise drop set** Level 3 do 1 set of 10–12 rm until fatigued, then drop to 75% of the initial weight and repeat until complete overload is achieved.

level			
repetitions	-	-	10–12 rm

thighs

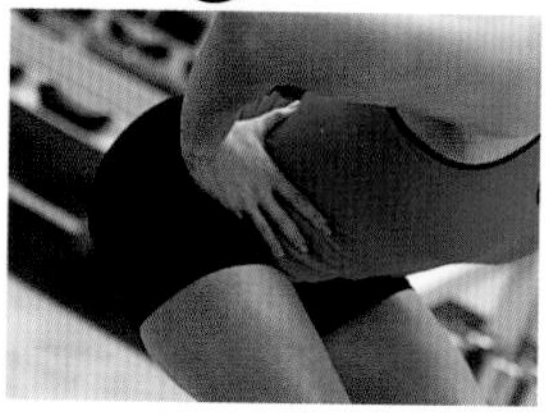

5 ◀ **Squat** Push through so you concentrate the weight of your body on your heels, as if you were sitting on an imaginary chair. **For squats, see page 80.**

level			
repetitions	14–16 rm	12–14 rm	10–12 rm

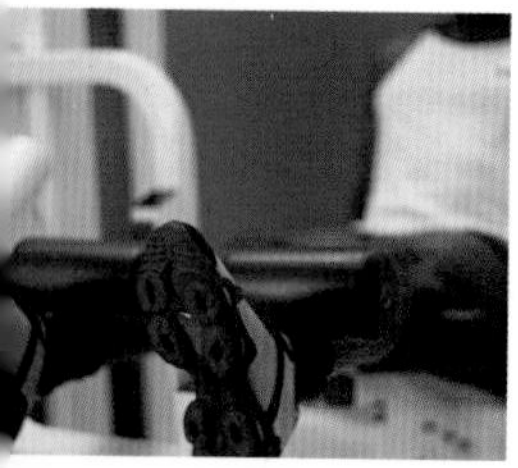

6 ◀ **Leg extension** Keep your abdominals tight and your lower back supported. **For leg extensions, see page 78.**

level			
repetitions	12 rm	14 rm	16 rm

7 ▶ **Power lunge** Push through the heel of the foot as you "spring" back to the start position. **For power lunges, see page 95.**

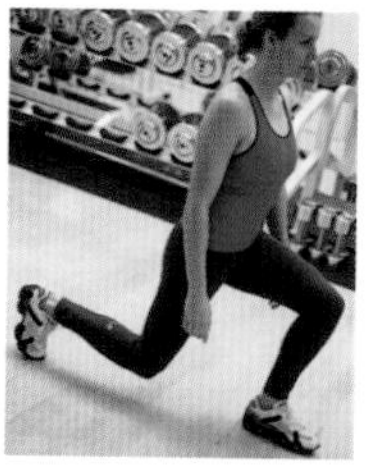

level			
repetitions	12	14	16

8 ▼ **Squat drop set** Level 3 do 10–12 rm, then drop to 75% weight and repeat until fatigued.

level			
repetitions	-	-	10–12 rm

triceps

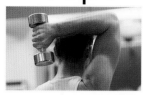

9 ◄ **Tricep overheads** Keep your elbow close to your head; take care not to let it "drift" around as you extend your arm. **For tricep overheads, see page 85.**

10 ► **Tricep extensions** Maintain good posture throughout by keeping your abdominals tight – this provides a stable base for the exercise. **For tricep extensions, see page 85.**

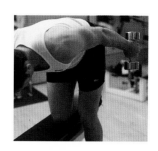

level			
repetitions	16 rm each arm	14 rm each arm	12 rm each arm

level			
repetitions	16 rm each arm	14 rm each arm	12 rm each arm

dips

This highly effective exercise concentrates work on the triceps.

level			
repetitions	14–16 rm	12–14 rm	10–12 rm

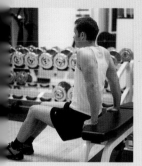

11 ◄ Place feet hip-width apart; keep your back straight and close to the bench.

► Slowly lower yourself down until your arms are bent at 90°, then push back up until arms are straight, but not locked.

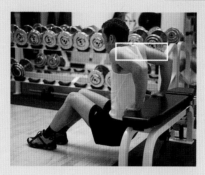

12 ▼ **Tricep overhead drop set** Level 3 do 10–12 rm, then drop to 75% weight and continue until overload.

level			
repetitions	-	-	12 rm each arm

biceps

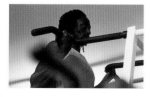

13 ▼ **Pull-up** Hold your abdominals tight to help maintain good posture. **For pull-ups, see page 83.**

level			
repetitions	14–16	12–14	10–12

14 ► **Single arm row** Keep your body stable as you pull the dumbbell toward your chest. **For single arm row, see page 86.**

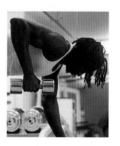

level			
repetitions	16 rm each arm	14 rm each arm	12 rm each arm

16 ► **Bicep curl drop set** Rest briefly, then level 3 do 10–12 rm, then do a drop set at 75% of the initial weight.

15 ► **Bicep curl** Squeeze your shoulder blades together as you perform this exercise. **For bicep curls, see page 84.**

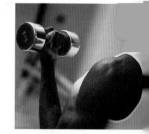

level			
repetitions	16 rm each arm	14 rm each arm	12 rm each arm

level			
repetitions	-	-	12 rm each arm

retest yourself

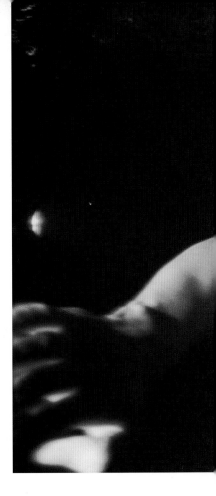

You have completed Phase Five and finished the program. You should be feeling stronger, leaner, and more flexible. Your improved level of fitness gives you the physical and emotional strength to achieve your goals and to feel better than ever before.

the payoff

The first two phases of the program helped you to create a good base of fitness – a stable foundation that would enable you to rise to the greater physical challenges ahead. Having worked through the last three phases of the plan, you have achieved the fitness of an advanced exerciser, whatever level you have been working at.

If you were not already, you are now familiar with a whole range of exercises that work the upper and lower body and test the heart and lungs. Circuits that combine resistance training and aerobic training have helped you to build stamina by working you at varying paces. Your aerobic capacity will have improved greatly. As a result, your metabolic rate will have increased, and, in most cases, your body will be burning energy at a faster rate than ever before.

You have worked up to – and are now comfortable with – more intensive methods of resistance training where you work with heavier weights but perform fewer repetitions. Your muscles should be more defined and your body more athletic in appearance.

Having developed a higher level of overall fitness, pyramid training has helped to sculpt your body. Compound training has helped to strengthen and tone specific muscle areas. If you have been exercising at level three, you have also used drop sets to get the most out of exercises to which your body may already be accustomed. By introducing variety to your exercise regime, you have overloaded your muscles and continued to challenge your body.

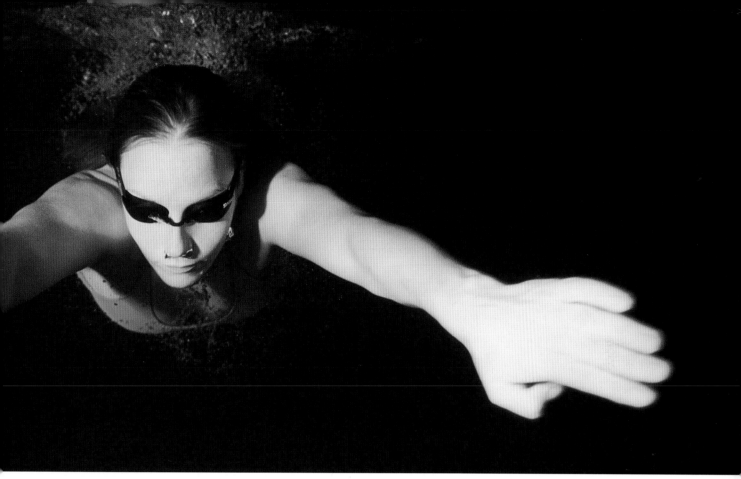

you feel stronger and leaner

the ultimate reward

Along with the nutritional goals that you have achieved, you have given your body all of the physical and nutritional support that it needs to function at optimum efficiency. You should feel the difference, both physically and mentally.

Your outlook on life should be brighter and your attitude more positive. You should feel more confident and much more capable. You find it easier to keep things in perspective and you manage stress well. It is not uncommon for me to take a client through the program and then hear about resulting successes in their professional lives. Other people notice when you feel better about yourself. You may want to make changes in your personal life – this is the time to do it.

Assess yourself continuously so you can track your progress. You bring about many positive changes as a result of completing the program, but the ultimate reward is the way that you feel about yourself.

summary

You will have worked hard to complete the program, but hopefully, you have also achieved personal goals along the way. Now is the time to set a new plan of action.

aim high

The program will have introduced substantial lifestyle changes for many people in terms of diet and exercise, and the way that you think about yourself. You may be surprised by the extent to which your body has changed, and it is very likely that you have a new and more positive outlook on life as well. You have made dramatic changes to your body's biochemical makeup, which will empower you and help you to aim for and achieve more ambitious goals in the future.

next steps

The plan does not end just because the book does. Over the past 90 days you have experienced the positive benefits of looking after your body. You have learned how to listen to and respond to your body's needs and treat it accordingly. Go and celebrate. Do something that you have been wanting to do for the past 90 days, but have been denying yourself. You should not constantly deprive yourself; it will only have the effect of making you crave those things more.

Take a break from the plan. Don't exercise for a week. Don't worry about your diet. After four days, start planning your next steps. Write down a new set of goals. The program has helped you to learn about your body's strengths and weaknesses, and you can set future goals with these in mind. You can repeat the program up to four times a year. Be creative. Look at areas of your life that you would like to change, and invariably there will be a health goal you can set that can help you achieve whatever that change may be. It is exciting to have completed the program, but it will be even more exciting to begin a new one.

changing body, changing demands

With your newfound fitness and self-confidence come new possibilities and an increasing desire to test yourself further. The healthier you become, the more obvious your next challenge will be to you. As you meet fresh challenges, you will begin to understand more about how your body responds to being tested in different ways, and your diet and exercise regimes will reflect this increased awareness. When once you might have been happy to complete a 45-minute aerobic workout, you may now feel ready to trek a mountain range. As your fitness and energy levels increase, you will have noticed the benefits of a diet that fuels your body efficiently. Your body will find it more difficult to cope with junk food than before, and increasing your intake of fat and sugar will impair your performance noticeably. Hopefully, realizations such as this will prevent you from slipping back into bad habits.

a word of warning

Having completed the plan, your improved level of fitness and health can leave you feeling better than you have felt in years, which is a wonderful thing, of course. However, you do need to be aware of your new strength – it can be potentially dangerous if you then approach a sport or activity with overenthusiastic vigor. I have seen people return to a sport that they have not played for some time and play so enthusiastically that the body cannot cope. It is usually the joints that suffer as a result of overexertion, but injuries such as tennis elbow are common among people who have regained a new vitality but have not yet learned to control it. Give your body time to adjust to the physical demands that a sport makes on it, and be aware of your limitations. There is nothing more frustrating than sustaining an injury that prevents you from exercising when you have worked hard to reach a higher level of fitness. I would not wish that on anyone.

133

monitoring yourself

To get the most from your training program, it is important to challenge the body continuously. Recording the progress that you make will help to keep you on track and motivated. It will also highlight your strengths and make you aware of any areas that may need extra work.

keeping a training diary

The program has encouraged you to push yourself as you have worked toward new and more challenging goals that were set at each one of the five phases. The different training techniques and intensities that you have worked at have tested your body in many ways, and it should be responding by developing and becoming stronger. If you have been following the program closely, you will have made steady progress toward a higher level of fitness.

After each workout, record the details of the session in a training diary. Write down the exercise you did, the weight you used, and the number of repetitions and sets that you performed. Since the program uses repetition maximums (RMs) in the resistance training, as you get in better shape you have to use more weight to keep achieving overload in the specified RMs. Remember, with resistance training, simply doing the required repetitions is not enough. To get results, you should feel that you are having to really push yourself to finish the last few repetitions in any set. This way you will continue to see the improvements that you strive for and which keep you motivated.

Keep a record of the length of your aerobic workout, your heart rate while exercising, and how you felt after each phase of the workout. Your exercise level in the program is determined by your heart rate.

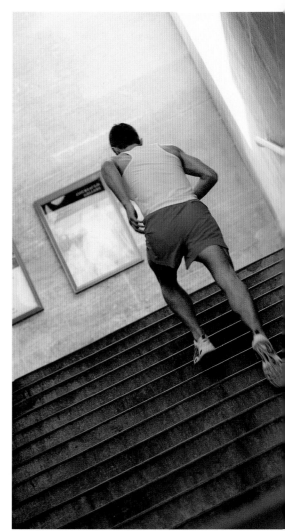
work toward bigger goals

As you get in better shape you will have to work harder to get your heart rate into the set target zones.

This detailed record of your progress throughout the program is the best way to monitor your development. It will ensure that you do the right amount of exercise each week and that you do not repeat the same routine too often with the result that your rate of progress drops. Remember that the key to good results is to vary your training methods constantly and to aim to improve your times and increase your weights each time you exercise.

Once you have finished this program, you can use your training diary to tailor a new program to your needs. Do not rely on your gym to set the speed at which you develop. Take the initiative yourself, and you will find that you progress much more quickly.

progress to a higher level of fitness

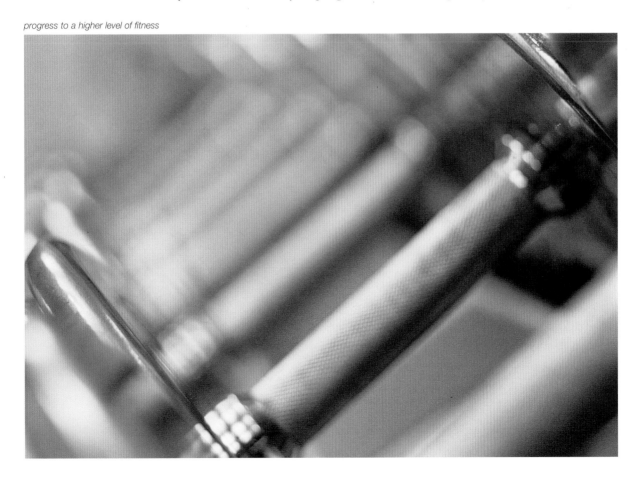

compiling a nutritional diary

Once you have completed the nutritional plan, the next objective is to keep up all that good work. The best way to do this is to keep a nutritional diary.

Once a month, choose three days, ideally two weekdays and either a Saturday or a Sunday, and write down everything that you eat and drink. To get an accurate overview of your diet, you must write down every single thing. We remember meals – breakfast, lunch, and dinner – but we often conveniently forget the snacks, extra cups of coffee, or afterwork alcoholic drink.

Your diary will enable you to check how close you are to the 80/20 percent diet balance ideal. Remember, 80 percent of the time you should be adhering to the nutritional goals as set out in the plan (*see page 114*), and the other 20 percent of the time you should be eating the foods that you enjoy, but which are not in the plan.

If your diet does not work out to be 80/20, set yourself some new nutritional goals for the month ahead. You might resolve to drink more water or to stop snacking on chocolate in the afternoon, for example.

It might help to write down the time of day that you eat or drink each thing, and how you felt before and after it. This will tell you whether you are eating and snacking at the right times of day, and also highlight any reactions your body may have to a particular food or drink. If, for example, you felt very tired before you ate lunch and found it difficult to concentrate, it could mean that you ate too late, did not have a good enough breakfast, or did not snack wisely mid-morning. Keeping a nutritional diary helps you to monitor what you eat and to adapt your diet accordingly.

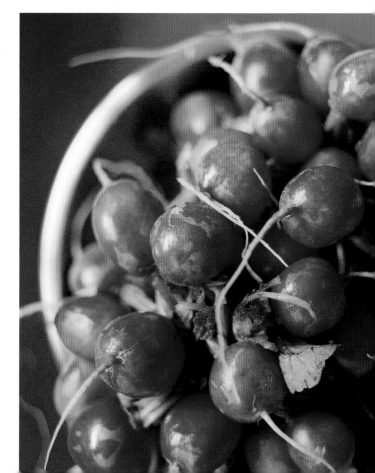

questionnaire results

physical questionnaire score

Your result gives you your level of fitness on a scale of one to three with three being the most advanced. The program will work best for you if you exercise at the level most suited to your ability.

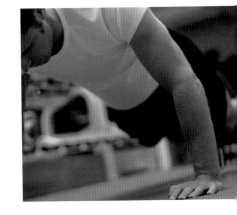

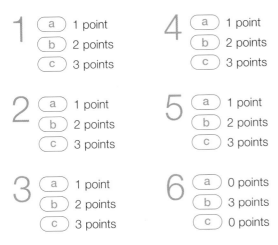

1
(a) 1 point
(b) 2 points
(c) 3 points

4
(a) 1 point
(b) 2 points
(c) 3 points

2
(a) 1 point
(b) 2 points
(c) 3 points

5
(a) 1 point
(b) 2 points
(c) 3 points

3
(a) 1 point
(b) 2 points
(c) 3 points

6
(a) 0 points
(b) 3 points
(c) 0 points

A score of between 5 and 8 points indicates the need for some serious changes to your lifestyle. You should follow the program at fitness level one. This level of fitness is probably the result of having ignored your fitness and health needs for many years. Be honest with yourself and use the program as a turning point. There are problems that you need to address, but the program can help you; it will transform the quality of your life.

A score of between 6 and 13 points indicates an average level of fitness. You should follow the program at fitness level two. You have probably being doing some form of exercise fairly regularly. Embarking upon the program now will reduce the likelihood of experiencing health problems later on in life.

A score of between 14 and 18 points indicates a high level of fitness. You should follow the program at fitness level three. You are quite focused and have almost certainly been physically active on a regular basis for some time. The program can help to keep you on track and prepare you for specific goals.

nutrition questionnaire score

Your total score gives an indication of how efficiently your digestive system functions and how acid or alkaline your body is. The more alkaline your body the better; the nutritional goals in the program guide toward a more alkaline diet.

1
- a) 3 points
- b) 2 points
- c) 1 point

2
- a) 3 points
- b) 2 points
- c) 1 point

3
- a) 3 points
- b) 2 points
- c) 1 point

4
- a) 3 points
- b) 2 points
- c) 1 point

5
- a) 3 points
- b) 2 points
- c) 1 point

6
- a) 3 points
- b) 2 points
- c) 1 point

7
- a) 3 points
- b) 2 points
- c) 1 point

8
- a) 3 points
- b) 2 points
- c) 1 point

9
- a) 3 points
- b) 2 points
- c) 1 point

10
- a) 3 points
- b) 2 points
- c) 1 point

11
- a) 3 points
- b) 2 points
- c) 1 point

12
- a) 3 points
- b) 2 points
- c) 1 point

13
- a) 3 points
- b) 2 points
- c) 1 point

14
- a) 3 points
- b) 2 points
- c) 1 point

15
- a) 3 points
- b) 0 points

16
- a) 3 points
- b) 2 points
- c) 1 point

17
- a) 3 points
- b) 2 points
- c) 1 point

18
- a) 3 points
- b) 2 points
- c) 1 point

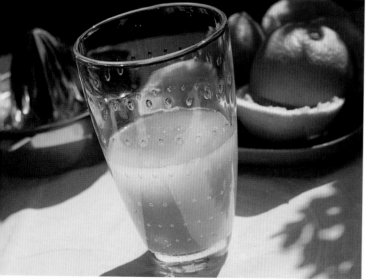

orange juice is slightly acidic

A total of 22 points or less indicates a good acid/alkaline balance in the body. **If your total comes to more than 23 points**, you have an acid-forming body and you should increase your intake of alkaline food *(see pages 70–1)*. **If you score more than 40 points**, a more alkaline diet and exercise program will have a radical effect on your quality of life.

personality questionnaire score

Your result allows you to categorize yourself loosely as either a type A personality, who is typically ambitious, focused, and more prone to stress, and a type B personality, who is more stable and relaxed.

exercise can help stress levels

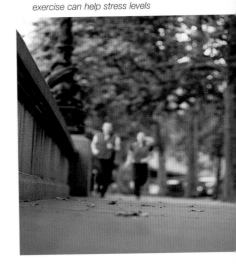
exercise can help stress levels

1
(a) 3 points
(b) 0 points

2
(a) 3 points
(b) 0 points

3
(a) 3 points
(b) 0 points

4
(a) 3 points
(b) 0 points

5
(a) 3 points
(b) 0 points

6
(a) 0 points
(b) 3 points

7
(a) 0 points
(b) 3 points

8
(a) 0 points
(b) 3 points

9
(a) 3 points
(b) 0 points

10
(a) 0 points
(b) 3 points

11
(a) 3 points
(b) 0 points

12
(a) 3 points
(b) 0 points

13
(a) 3 points
(b) 0 points

A score of 18 points or more indicates a type A personality. You have a tendency toward an acid-forming body, which may be more prone to toxin buildup. Try to follow a more alkaline-forming diet and exercise aerobically. Take time out to escape the pressures of work; meditation, yoga, natural therapies, or a pastime that takes you outdoors in a relaxed environment would all be good additions to your workout program. Spend time every other day doing a stretching routine (*see pages 46–7*). Breathe deeply during stretching. This encourages oxygen to flow freely around the body and to the brain.

A score of 15 points indicates tendencies toward both type A and type B personalities. Stick to an alkaline diet. You probably cope quite well with stress.

A score of 12 points or less indicates a type B personality. You probably have a less acid-forming body, which is less prone to toxin buildup. Keep your water intake high and eat plenty of fresh fruit and vegetables to assist digestion and sustain energy levels. You manage stress well.

terminology

Below is a list of terms used throughout this book, each of which is followed by a definition. Where a term, used as part of a definition, has its own full entry, that term is displayed in *italics*.

aerobic capacity
The body's ability to take in and utilize oxygen. *Aerobic exercise* increases aerobic capacity.

aerobic exercise
Exercise "with oxygen"; it builds heart and lung strength and enhances the body's ability to take in oxygen, feed oxygenated blood around the body, and create energy. The long-term effects of aerobic exercise are lower blood pressure, decreased risk of heart problems, and better circulation. It also helps to fight the onset and effects of aging.

abdominals
These are the muscles of the stomach area. The muscle group extends from the rib cage to the pelvis and comprises three main muscles of importance: the rectus abdominus (the "six pack" muscles that run down the middle of the stomach), the obliques (the muscles on the outside of the stomach area), and the quadratus lumborum (the deep muscle that wraps around the mid-section of the torso and is important for posture).

anaerobic exercise
Exercise "without oxygen"; fast explosive work that cannot be sustained for long periods of time. This form of exercise uses the less efficient anaerobic energy system that can be maintained for only short bursts.

antioxidants
The collective name given to the nutrients and other substances that fight the buildup of *free radicals*.

body mass index (BMI)
A good indicator of whether body size is in proportion to body structure. It measures weight in relation to frame size, taking into account total weight and body fat.

basal metabolic rate (BMR)
The rate at which the body burns calories. Exercise will increase the body's BMR so that it burns more calories even when inactive. Dieting lowers the BMR, making body management much harder.

biceps
The muscles at the front of the upper arms; used to bend the arms.

circuit training
A training method where a series of exercises is performed, each for a short period of time. Circuit training can tone the muscles as well as having a heart-conditioning effect.

constant pace training
A form of cardiovascular training that requires the heart rate being raised to the ideal level and then being maintained at that level for a specified period of time.

deltoids
The three muscles of the shoulders, used in raising the arms up to the sides.

drop set
A weight training method where you fatigue the muscles, then drop the resistance to 75 percent of the first weight and continue until the muscle is fatigued once again.

free radicals
The naturally occurring rogue oxygen molecules that roam around the body destroying cells. Poor diet, stress, and lack of exercise increase the buildup of free radicals. Many of the foods recommended in the book's nutritional program are aimed at fighting the buildup of free radicals.

glutes
The muscles of the butt and hip area, which are used in the action of moving the leg backward.

hamstrings
The muscles at the backs of the thighs; used to bend the legs.

hip flexor
The muscles of the hip area; they are used in the action of bringing the knee up to the chest or raising the knee.

hip-to-waist ratio
A figure that is arrived at by dividing the measurement of the hip by the measurement of the waist; used to assess a person's health in relation to their body fat distribution.

interval training
A cardiovascular training method that works the heart within the *optimum training zone*. It works the heart in the higher range of the training zone, then uses the lower range as a recovery period; builds cardiovascular endurance.

lats / latissimus dorsi
The large muscle of the back, which is used in all actions pulling down and toward the body.

maximum heart rate (MHR)
The maximum level to which a person should raise their heart rate; it is determined by age and calculated in beats per minute (bpm).

omega-3 fatty acid
The essential fatty acid found in oily fish. Excellent for the body, helps build healthy cells, aids in the production of energy, and is an important *antioxidant*.

omega-6 fatty acid
The healthy oil found in olives, nuts, and seeds; essential for the healthy maintenance of the body.

optimum training zone
The age-related heart rate training range that is ideal for burning fat and building cardiovascular strength; usually between 75 and 90 percent of *maximum heart rate*.

overloading
The process of pushing the body beyond its usual physical limits, which helps to achieve greater results when exercising. You should aim to achieve overload whenever you work out.

pectorals
The muscles of the chest area, used in moving the arms forward and pushing away from the body.

peripheral heart action (PHA)
A resistance training technique that also conditions the heart. It concentrates exercises on the upper and lower body alternately, so the heart has to work hard to pump blood to the muscles at both ends of the body.

pronation / pronate
With reference to the foot, this is a tendency to walk with body weight concentrated on the insides of the feet; shoes tend to wear on the inner sides of the soles. Wearing shoes suitable for your feet when exercising can help correct a tendency toward pronation.

pyramid training
A training method that makes the body work harder with every set of exercises, therefore *overloading* the body to achieve greater improvement.

quads / quadriceps
The muscles of the fronts of the thighs, used to straighten the legs.

repetition (rep)
In *resistance training* a rep is one complete performance of an exercise, moving from the start position and back to the finish position. If you are asked to do 14 reps of an exercise, you should repeat that exercise 14 times before stopping.

repetition maximum (RM)
The number of *repetitions* of a particular exercise to be performed to achieve *overload* on the muscles.

resistance training
A training method that uses weights to tone and build the muscles.

saturated fat
Oil and fat that is solid at room temperature; found in meat products and chemically processed foods. The unhealthiest form of fat, it has been linked to high blood pressure and heart disease.

set
The number of repetitions you perform of an exercise at one time, without pausing. You are often asked to repeat sets, in which case you can take a short rest period between each set.

supination / supinate
With reference to the foot, this is a tendency to walk with body weight concentrated on the outsides of the feet; shoes tend to wear on the outer sides of the soles. Wearing shoes suitable for your feet when exercising can help correct a tendency toward supination.

unsaturated fat
Oil, such as olive oil, and fat that is liquid at room temperature; found in fish, nuts, seeds, and grains. The healthiest form of fat, it is essential for many of the functions of the body.

index

acknowledgments

author's acknowledgments

I would like to thank Mary-Clare Jerram and all at DK who made writing my debut book a possibility and who, along the way, have made the whole process greatly entertaining.

Thank you to the photographic dynamic duo of Reuben ("I want it to be organic!") Paris and Janeanne ("I'm not hungover, I come from Scotland, this is normal for the morning!"), who between them have produced the moodiest series of photos for a fitness book I have ever seen.

Thank you to Tracy Killick in particular who, in the line of duty, provided those present with a foretaste of her gymnastic prowess, performing a double back flip and in the process very kindly donating one of her ribs to the greater cause of the book – great cabaret for a wet day on a London roof! The book looks amazing, Tracy! Thank you.

Thanks to Queen Nasim who has spent many hours trawling through text on exercise, diet, and lifestyle. She thankfully displayed great patience and stopped short of turning into Prince Naseem with me when I was pushing to reach a deadline!

Special thanks to two of my training team, Lucy and Drako, who provided their time and their bodies to the project. Lucy caused problems for the underwater photographer by swimming so fast that the film could barely keep up! Drako provided his anatomical study model body for many of the exercises, and is so laid-back he often needs waking up! Thank you both for your time and effort; it has been greatly appreciated.

Thank you to Ralph Lauren, in particular to Helen Young and to Emer Melody, for providing the clothing for the book. They provide us with fantastic ongoing support at all times. I advise everyone to go out and buy their clothes!

Big thanks to my brother, Jon, who also appears in the book (he is the one who looks a bit like me only older!!), and who I have worked closely with to produce the research and text for the book. I know it's a family thing to work hard together on projects, but it often goes beyond the call of duty (this particularly applies when being soaked with water on a cold day for the sake of a photo!).

For anyone else who has been involved with the production of this book in any way I give my thanks. I would go on to mention more, but this is in danger of becoming a bit "Oscar" gushy so I'll quit while I'm ahead!
Matt

publisher's acknowledgments

Dorling Kindersley would like to thank Andrew Bell for underwater photography; Polo Sport for kindly supplying clothing from their new RLX range; One Aldwych and Royal Garden Hotel for the use of their facilities; Irene Lyford and Lesley Malkin for editorial assistance; Ros Saunders, Karen Sawyer, and William Walton for design assistance. Thanks to Paul Reid at Cobalt for concept design. Thanks to models Lucy Arrowsmith, Drako Mkpa, Caroline Wildman, Rebecca Lewis, Helen Thomas, Matt Roberts, and Jon Roberts.

Matt Roberts gyms can be found at:

matt roberts personal training
32–4 Jermyn Street
London SW1Y 6HS
England
Tel: +44 20 7491 4232
Fax: +44 20 7491 4233

matt roberts at one
One Aldwych
London WC2B 4BZ
England
Tel: +44 20 7300 0600
Fax: +44 20 7300 0601

matt roberts at le saint géran
Poste de Flacq
île Maurice
Tel: +33 (230) 401 1000
Fax: +33 (230) 401 1111

matt roberts at the royal garden
2–24 Kensington High Street
London W8 4PT
England
Tel: +44 20 7361 1994/5
Fax: +44 20 7361 1991

Matt Roberts is developing his own line of health- and fitness-related products. For a list of products and recommended retailers, contact the head office at:

matt roberts personal training
lower basement
47 Albermarle Street
London W1X 3FE
England
Tel: +44 20 7937 7722